# USING GROUNDED THEORY IN NURSING

**Rita Sara Schreiber, RN, DNS,** is an Associate Professor at the School of Nursing, University of Victoria in British Columbia, Canada. With her colleagues, she is founder of the Grounded Theory Club, a mentoring project to enable grounded theorists to develop their own research skills as well as the methodology. She has published multiple peer-reviewed articles and book chapters in areas of practice, gender, methodology, and women's experience with depression and treatment.

**Phyllis Noerager Stern, DNS, FAAN, NAP**, holds the position of Professor and Glenn W. Irwin, Jr., MD Research Scholar at the School of Nursing, and a joint appointment in Women's Studies at Indiana University, Indianapolis, Indiana. She is Editor-in-Chief of the interdisciplinary refereed journal, *Health Care for Women International,* and Council General (CEO) and co-founder of the International Council on Women's Health Issues. She holds a charter membership in the Grounded Theory Institute.

# USING GROUNDED THEORY IN NURSING

**RITA SARA SCHREIBER,** RN, DNS
**PHYLLIS NOERAGER STERN,** DNS, FAAN, NAP

EDITORS

 SPRINGER PUBLISHING COMPANY

Springer Publishing Company, Inc.
536 Broadway
New York, NY 10012-3955

*Acquisitions Editor: Ruth Chasek*
*Production Editor: J. Hurkin-Torres*
*Cover design by Susan Hauley*

02 03 04 05 / 5 4 3 2

---

**Library of Congress Cataloging-in-Publication Data**

Using grounded theory in nursing/Rita Sara Schreiber, Phyllis Noerager Stern, editors.
    p. ; cm.
  Includes bibliographical references and index.
  ISBN 0-8261-1406-7
  1. Nursing—Research.  2. Grounded theory.  I. Schreiber, Rita Sara.  II. Stern, Phyllis Noerager.
  [DNLM: 1. Nursing Research—methods. WY 20.5 U838 2001]
  RT81.5 .U83 2001
  610.73'07'2—dc21
                                                  00-067952
                                                              CIP

---

Printed in the United States of America by Maple-Vail

To Barney and Anselm, who gave us so much to debate about
and who challenged us to think beyond the boundaries

# Contents

# Contributors

**Sheila McGuire Bunting, PhD, RN,** is an Associate Professor of Nursing in the Department of Community Nursing, Medical College of Georgia. She has many years of experience in nursing practice and in teaching community health nursing as well as research and theory to graduate and undergraduate students. Her research interests and the topics of her publications include care of persons with HIV disease and their families, decision-making in health care, and feminism in nursing.

**Eleanor Krassen Covan, PhD,** is the Director of Gerontology Programs at the University of North Carolina at Wilmington. She holds the position of Professor of Sociology in the Department of Sociology and Criminal Justice. Her research interests include the social psychology of elder persons, caregiving networks within the context of culture, and the social structural processes that impact on intergenerational relationships. She has a strong eclectic background in sociological research methods. Most recently, she has been investigating the impact of natural disasters on the elderly in southeastern North Carolina.

**Claire Burke Draucker, RN, PhD, CS,** is an Associate Professor in the College of Nursing, Kent State University. She is a licensed psychologist in the state of Ohio and a Certified Clinical Specialist in Psychiatric Mental Health Nursing. Dr. Draucker has conducted studies on early family experiences and later victimization in the lives of women, the healing processes of women and men who were sexually abused as children, and women's responses to sexual violence by male intimates. She is the author of *Counseling Adult Survivors of Childhood Sexual Abuse.*

**Wendy Hall, RN, PhD**, is an Associate Professor at the School of Nursing, University of British Columbia. She earned her BN from the University of Manitoba, her MSN from the University of British Columbia, and her PhD from the University of Manchester. Her research has focused on the transition to parenting and has included a number of grounded theory studies. Dr. Hall developed the Role Enactment Questionnaire from two grounded theory studies, one with women in dual-earner couples, the other with men with infants in dual-earner couples.

**Margaret H. Kearney, PhD, RNC,** is a women's health nurse practitioner and an Associate Professor of Nursing at Boston College in Chestnut Hill, Massachusetts. She studied grounded theory technique with Anselm Strauss at the University of California at San Francisco and has conducted a number of studies with addicted and recovering women using the grounded theory approach. Her current qualitative and quantitative research focuses on the impact of violence during pregnancy, nursing support of socially high-risk pregnant women and mothers, and addiction recovery in homeless men. She has published two grounded formal theories and has recently completed a third formal theory analysis of women's experiences of domestic violence.

**Marjorie MacDonald, RN, PhD,** is an Assistant Professor at the School of Nursing, University of Victoria. She has a PhD in Interdisciplinary Studies in Health Promotion from the University of British Columbia. Her research and practice focus is on community and public health nursing with specific interests in school and adolescent health, particularly related to alcohol, tobacco, and other drug use. She also has a background in health policy and program evaluation. With her colleagues, Dr. MacDonald is a co-founder of the Grounded Theory Club.

**Caroline Mallory, RN, PhD,** completed doctoral studies at Indiana University in Indianapolis and postdoctoral study at the School of Nursing, University of North Carolina at Chapel Hill, where she was selected to receive Institutional and Individual National Research Service Awards from the National Institute of Health. Her research is related to prevention of HIV/AIDS among women marginalized by poverty, drug use, and survival sex. Presently, Dr. Mallory is an Assistant Professor at Mennonite College of Nursing at Illinois State University in Normal, Illinois.

**Katharyn Antle May, RN, PhD,** is a Professor and Dean at the School of Nursing, University of Wisconsin in Madison, Wisconsin. She earned her BSN from Duke University and her MSN and DNSc from the University of California, San Francisco School of Nursing, where she studied grounded theory method with Anselm Strauss, Leonard Schatzman, and Phyllis Stern. Her research has focused on the psychosocial transition of pregnancy and childbirth, including a three-year grounded theory study on the effects of preterm labor management on families, a project funded by the National Institute for Nursing Research.

**Marilyn Merritt-Gray, BN, MN,** is an Associate Professor in the Faculty of Nursing, University of New Brunswick, Canada. She has extensive experience as a community mental health nurse in rural Atlantic Canada. She completed her graduate work at the University of Washington in Psychosocial Nursing. The bulk of her research has been collaborative, focussing on woman abuse from a survivor and wellness perspective, rural health care policy and service delivery issues, and community development practice.

**P. Jane Milliken, RN, PhD,** is an Assistant Professor of Nursing at the University of Victoria. Her BSc in Nursing and her MA and PhD in sociology were all received from the University of Alberta. This combination of nursing and sociology reflects her research interests in the social causes and consequences of chronic illness as well as aging and mental health. Her most recent work focuses on the effects of schizophrenia upon families. With her colleagues, Dr. Milliken is a co-founder of the Grounded Theory Club.

**Janice M. Morse, PhD (Nurs), PhD (Anthro), D.Nurs (Hon),** is the Director of the International Institute for Qualitative Methodology and Professor, Faculty of Nursing, University of Alberta. She has published extensively in the areas of comfort, suffering, and qualitative methods, and serves as editor of the bi-monthly, international, interdisciplinary journal, *Qualitative Health Research.*

**Suzanne Pursley-Crotteau, PhD, RN, CS, CARN,** is a nurse researcher, educator, and clinician. Her research interests are in the areas of women's mental health (including substance use) and consumer adaptation to telehealth technology, using qualitative methods. Dr. Pursley-Crotteau is presently the Supervisory Human Subjects Protection Scientist for the Office of Regulation and Compliance and Quality Control, Army Surgeon General in Frederick, Maryland.

**Judith Wuest, MN, PhD,** is a Professor in the Faculty of Nursing at the University of New Brunswick in Fredericton, New Brunswick, Canada. She is also affiliated with the Muriel McQueen Fergusson Centre for Family Violence Research. Her research interests are in women's caregiving and woman abuse, using feminist grounded theory and participatory research approaches. She and her colleagues presently hold funding from the Medical Research Council of Canada and the National Health Research and Development Program to study health promotion processes in single parent families who have experienced woman abuse and the effects of public policy on these processes.

# Preface

We conceived this book during chats in the hallways at several conferences, most notably the 1997 meetings of the International Council of Nurses in Vancouver, British Columbia. It was at that conference that we, along with our colleagues Dauna Crooks and Cynthia Ricci McCloskey, conducted a symposium on grounded theory and women's health, two of our passions. We were pleased at the considerable excitement in the crowded lecture hall about doing grounded theory research. For us it was a watershed experience to see this critical mass of scholars who shared our enthusiasm about the method. It was evident to us that there is a growing interest among nurses in conducting grounded theory research, and from their multiple queries, we saw the need for a source book where scholars could go for illumination.

At about the same time, a handful of faculty members and graduate students at the University of Victoria School of Nursing began to meet regularly in what eventually became known as the Grounded Theory Club (GTC). This was, in part, an effort to provide a place for exploration of the method and some of the epistemological and methodological challenges involved in conducting grounded theory research. One of the activities of GTC members involves sharing resources and references. After several months, it became clear to us that most of the available published literature failed to reflect grounded theory as some of the GTC members thought we understood and used it. This was particularly problematic for students new to the method who sought clear direction and advice to guide their studies. Members of the GTC, along with other North American long-term and newer, more questioning scholars, came together to bring forth our collective understanding and wisdom in the clearest possible format.

To begin the process, we took a page from Jan Morse and decided to hold a two-day seminar, bringing together the contributing authors in Victoria, British Columbia, in January 1999. It was a time for authors to meet (or reacquaint themselves with) each other and have some fairly intense formal and informal discussions about the challenges and rewards of doing grounded theory research. During the scheduled meeting times, each draft chapter was opened for critique, and members of the group offered suggestions for improvement, resources, and references, and provided other perspectives as well as some support. Plans were made for how to review manuscripts at later stages of development. Since the Victoria meeting, updated (and some new) manuscripts flew back and forth between and among authors and editors via the electronic ether.

This text represents our attempt to identify and raise questions about grounded theory and how it is currently used in nursing research. We have brought together nursing researchers conducting, and reflecting on, grounded theory as a research method. As the reader will note, there are some conflicting views on the same issues expressed by different authors in this text. In our view, scholarly discussion is a positive process in attempting to resolve the issues and controversies surrounding grounded theory research. Thus, we highlight some key challenges researchers must consider as they conduct their inquiries.

*Rita Sara Schreiber*
*Phyllis Noerager Stern*

# Acknowledgments

We are grateful for the contributions of everyone who helped us in the conception, preparation, and production of this book. Dr. Martin Taylor, Dr. Anita Molzahn, and Dr. Janet Storch, all of the University of Victoria, provided space and invaluable support for the seminar of contributing authors back in the days when this book was still a glint in its parents' eyes. Ken Underdahl fed us imaginatively and well, and kept our spirits going through two long days of work. Dr. Dauna Crooks, Dr. Patricia Munhall, and Dr. Claire Draucker all offered their wise support and counsel at key stages throughout the process. Margo McCanney of the University of Victoria and Shannon McDonald of Indiana University-Purdue University at Indianapolis helped us in countless ways to overcome the challenges of technology. Dr. Mary Ann Jezewski first introduced Rita to grounded theory and oversaw her first study. Dr. Eleanor Covan got Phyllis started on the road to computer virus vaccinating. Our editor at Springer, Ruth Chasek, guided us through the publishing maze and provided wise, timely advice throughout. All of the authors in this book have collaborated diligently to provide thoughtful, scholarly review and critique of one another's chapters. We particularly thank Steven, Hope, and Paula for their patience and unending faith in us. These people made this book possible.

# Introduction

Grounded theory, a qualitative, inductive approach to research, was originally developed by Glaser and Strauss (1967) who "discovered" it as a way to help reveal how people manage the problematic situations in their lives. By directly observing and talking with people, researchers can now study how people make sense of their lives, particularly their health experiences, and use that understanding to resolve their challenges. The publication of *Discovery of Grounded Theory* (Glaser & Strauss, 1967) marked a dramatic breakthrough in nursing research by providing investigators with the tools to study health phenomena from the perspective of those experiencing them.

As a review of the literature and dissertation abstracts demonstrates, interest in qualitative methods in general and grounded theory in particular has burgeoned in the past 10 years. A review of CINAHL revealed that grounded theory is the second most popular qualitative research method published in nursing. Further, the majority of grounded theory dissertations have appeared in the past decade, and most of those have been within the past two years, indicating an exponential rise in interest in the method. Yet, the methodological writing on grounded theory has failed to keep pace with published findings. We, as both authors and editors, feel unsettled at the mismatch between what is written and our own understanding and practice of the method. This book represents an effort to raise awareness of the ontological and philosophical underpinnings of grounded theory and how these influence the way we conduct research.

Because grounded theory is an exploratory method of research, it does not begin from a position of an existing theory and pre-defined concepts. Rather, as the data, which can be anything, are collected, coded, and analyzed simultaneously, concepts and properties become evident (Glaser & Strauss, 1967). Grounded theory is sometimes referred to as the constant comparative method because every piece of coded data is compared with every other piece of data, with concepts and categories, and with all levels of abstraction as the developing theory begins to take form. At each stage of analysis, hypotheses or hunches are generated and tested against the data so that a core category and an explanatory theory of behavior arise from that data. However, we hope to make it clear that there is much more involved in doing grounded theory than just constant comparison.

We have found grounded theory to be the method of choice when we want to learn how people manage their lives in the context of existing or potential health challenges, and as such, is admirably suited to nursing inquiry. What is key in this process is learning the ways that people understand and deal with what is happening to them over time. Grounded theory was designed to reveal the human characteristic of change in response to (or anticipation of) various life circumstances. It is particularly useful for research in situations that have not been previously studied, where existing research has left major gaps, and where a new perspective might be desirable to identify areas for nursing intervention.

In generating this book, we gathered together a number of grounded theorists in both the U.S. and Canada representing a range of experiences with the method. With this mix, our plan was to create tension between traditional grounded theory as originally practiced and newer perspectives on the method. We believe we have succeeded in this goal.

What is different about this book is the broad coverage by the authors of the method and its background, as well as its ontological and epistemological roots and recent directions. The outcome of this background, mixed with authors who have little reserve when recording their points of view, is that the reader will find not all of our contributors agreeing with one another. Personally, we glory in academic debates, and our hope is that you, as reader, will be stimulated to do your own methodological investigations. We must confess that as editors *we* often disagree, but we view this debate as a healthy ingredient in a research environment.

We need to make the point, however, that we consider each chapter of this book as sound logic and creativity. The authors are true to grounded theory in its intent: to be a voice for the point of view of people who may not otherwise be heard and for the perspectives of participants on the way health professionals can learn to respect their chosen ways of solving life problems.

Finally, it has been our experience that everyone who uses grounded theory spins it to suit his or her way of thinking, just as everyone who reads a book takes away a somewhat different message. A word of caution here. The researcher using grounded theory needs to exercise care to avoid a departure from the intent of the authors who developed it, Glaser and Strauss. In short, there are a number of variations in doing grounded theory, all of which are acceptable. On the other hand, there are a lot of wrong ways of doing it. We hope we help you avoid those wrong ways.

## REFERENCE

Glaser, B. M., & Strauss, A. (1967). *The discovery of grounded theory.* Chicago, IL: Aldine.

# CHAPTER 1

# Situating Grounded Theory Within Qualitative Inquiry

**Janice M. Morse**

## SITUATING GROUNDED THEORY WITHIN QUALITATIVE INQUIRY

Grounded theory is a major qualitative method. In the three decades since its development, it has made a significant impact on the development of social science theory and, as this volume attests, is currently making a major contribution to nursing research. Despite the extensive use of grounded theory over the past 30 years and the publication of several landmark methodological textbooks, many issues pertaining to the purpose and use of grounded theory continue to remain unclear. In particular, there is a conspicuous silence about the appropriate application(s) of the grounded theory method and silence about when (and even if ever) it is inappropriately used. In this chapter, I will attempt to situate grounded theory within the domain of qualitative inquiry by exploring the characteristics and strengths of the theory method. In other words, I will consider methodologically, What does grounded theory do best?

Before beginning this discussion, however, two points must be made clear. The first is that there are two dominant schools of grounded theory that have emerged over recent years, that of Anselm Strauss and that of Barney Glaser (Melia, 1996; Stern, 1994), which immediately creates some tension in this discussion. Wherever necessary, the perspective of each of these schools of grounded theory will be addressed separately. The second point is that I will treat grounded theory as a method—that is, as a particular approach to analyze data that originally evolved through a particular theoretical perspective (i.e., symbolic interactionism). As such, it involves a unique perspective or way of conceptualizing reality using data (Strauss, 1987, p. 5), and particular strategies or techniques designed to meet analytic goals. Although data sources (and the forms of data) remain less clearly specified for grounded theory method ("all is data" [Glaser, 1998, p. 8]), the actual strategies used for data analysis are described in greater detail by grounded theorists than by methodologists for any other qualitative method. Thus, I will be treating grounded theory as a formal and mature qualitative method.

## Characteristics of Grounded Theory Research

Completed grounded theory projects have a distinct style and form, one that is easily recognizable as "a grounded theory" study. Distinguishing characteristics of grounded theory are: (a) grounded theory focuses on a process and trajectory, resulting in identifiable stages and phases; (b) it uses gerunds (Glaser, 1978, 1996) indicating action and change; (c) it has a core variable or category (Strauss & Corbin, 1998), a *Basic Social Process* or *Basic Social Psychological Process* (Glaser, 1978) that ties stages and phases of the theory together; and (d) grounded theory is abstract (as is all theory), but it is unique in that it makes the synthesis of descriptive data readily apparent through its concepts and relational statements. Thus, grounded theory is usually aimed at producing mid-range theories.

Can scientific results be labeled "grounded theory" without these characteristics? Probably not. Notwithstanding the researcher's claims about "doing" grounded theory, without these essential theoretical structures the study is not grounded theory, and certainly not a good grounded theory study.

## The Nature of Theory in Grounded Theory

The theory that is derived from grounded theory is typically a substantive mid-range theory. That is, it is most frequently focused on a behavioral concept, such as trust, resilience, caring, coping, and so forth, or on an interesting behavioral phenomenon. In early grounded theory method books (Glaser & Strauss, 1967), an inquiry into a concept or topic of interest was clearly described as a process with the resulting theory consisting of phases and stages. Such theory was built around a Basic Social Process (BSP) which comprises of either a Basic Social Psychological Process (BSPP) or a Basic Social Structural Process (BSSP) or core category (Glaser, 1978, p. 142; 1996, p. 135) or central category (Strauss & Corbin, 1998, p. 146). The BSP/BSPP is a central theme that unites all categories and explains most of the variation among the data. The trajectural nature of grounded theory is further constructed with concept labels identified as gerunds (labels ending in "-ing") (Glaser, 1996), and categories and concepts built by identifying "strategies" or "influencing factors." In fact, when listing grounded theories in nursing by "knowledge clusters," Benoleil (1996) uses these processes or influencing factors as subheadings, such as "Interventions and interactional processes by nurses" or "Psychological processes of vulnerable people."

How crucial is process to grounded theory?[1] Strauss and Corbin (1998) write:

> . . . bringing process into the analysis is essential. Process can be the organizing thread or central category of a theory, or it can take a less prominent role. Regardless of the role it plays, process can be thought of as the difference between a snapshot and a moving picture. . . Theory without process is missing a vital part of its story—how the action/interaction evolves. (p. 179)

They also add that:

[process is] a series of evolving sequences of action/interaction that occur over time and space, changing or sometimes remaining the

---

[1]Interestingly, in their Overview, Strauss and Corbin (1994) do not discuss process at all in the distinguishing features for grounded theory.

same in response to the situation or context. The action/interaction may be strategic, taken in response to problematic situations, or it may be quite routine. . . It may be orderly, interrupted, sequential, or coordinated—or in some cases a complete mess. What makes the action/interaction process is its evolving nature and its varying forms, rhythms, and pacing all related to some purpose. (p. 165)

How significant is *process* to grounded theory? Process implies a beginning and an end, an antecedent and a consequence, that is, some level of causality. Ideally, this means that in order to identify a trajectory, data should be temporal, similar to stories with a beginning, middle, and end. As opposed to "snippet data" (that is, data that is obtained in response to a question in a focus group or semi-structured interview), grounded theory data should be in a form by which the process and its structure can be readily identified. Therefore the narrative form, with events told as they unfold, is best suited for grounded theory data. Initially, participants who have experienced the phenomena or who have lived through the experience should be invited to "tell their stories" so that an overview of the process may be obtained. This structure then forms the sampling frame for purposely selecting other participants or structuring observations. Once the researcher has a broad overview of the process then sampling may be directed to transitions, critical junctures or significant points in the process, or observations targeted to significant events. Such strategies are the beginnings of theoretical sampling.

In this way, obtaining accounts of the whole event provides, at least, a preliminary understanding of the domain or of "what is going on." Comprehension (Morse, 1997) will thus be achieved earlier and faster than if the researcher worked prospectively, "going through" the experience with participants. This structure may facilitate the identification of the stages and phases; it may assist in the identification of critical junctures or points that may account for variation in data. At the very least, it provides the researcher with an important understanding of the context.

Can grounded theory be conducted using snippet data from focus groups or semi-structured questionnaires? These data are obtained from conversations and they rarely contain the continuous in-depth stories that the retrospective accounts from unstructured interviews do. The disjointedness of the data structure in focus group data makes incorporation of these data into grounded theory clumsy and slow. Therefore, these data are used to supplement data in particular areas once the basic structure has been identified on the basis of narratives.

The key to grounded theory is that psychosocial process is discoverable. This "process" is not simply the temporal linking of day-to-day events to construct the grounded theory itself. The theory that emerges is not obvious and doing grounded theory is not easy, simple or fast. Rather, it is the processes of analysis, the strategies and techniques of coding, categorizing, and re-categorizing, that place data in a form that enables the discovery of the BSP, BSPP, BSSP, the core variable or category.

## Theoretical Form

The fact that grounded theory is problem-focused and directed towards a process requires the theoretical structure be typically one of linked stages and phases. Categories identified in the data are developed as concepts and then linked as a trajectory. The theory is usually categorized as mid-range; while it is not usually obvious, it is also not complex; it is often diagrammed and organized around a central theme (basic processes or core variables/categories). Can the theory have two or more competing major basic processes or major core variables/categories? Perhaps, but this is rarely seen. The basic processes or core variables/categories appear to serve the purpose of focusing the researcher, so that a second set, if identified, is often poorly integrated into the theory. Perhaps, pushed by the pressure to publish on the basis of the same data, researchers sometimes use a second major core variable. Furthermore, if the basic processes or core variables/categories reveal a converse case (for instance, the ability to do . . . and the ability not to do . . . ), these two processes may be diagrammed as different processes, in different theoretical schemes, rather than expressed in the same model. For example, with Bottorff, I was required to develop two models of different structures to illustrate breast-feeding mothers' ability and inability to express breast milk (Morse & Bottorff, 1988). At first glance, these two processes should logically be integrated in the same model, however, it was elucidated that these two processes are, in fact, not opposing parts of the same phenomenon. The fact that the inability to express breast milk follows a different pattern than the ability to express (and the converse is not a mirror image of the first pattern), shows the value of grounded theory and the surprises that occur with its uses.

Focusing, while arguably essential for developing theory, has two ramifications. Firstly, it somewhat limits the explanatory value of the theory by keeping it narrow in scope. This is a mixed blessing. For students it ensures that their work remains manageable as a thesis or dissertation. On the other hand, it may also artificially restrict or simplify reality, thereby omitting processes that are significant or that transect the process under study. For example, hope is an important concept that assists individuals when emerging from suffering and likewise merges with the concept of suffering. But a grounded theory focusing on suffering would only address this junction—it would not necessarily explore hope as it did not relate to suffering. This could be resolved by exploring the topic more comprehensively through the use of multiple grounded theories or other techniques such as linking concepts (Morse & Penrod, 1999). Secondly, focusing on producing only one core variable keeps the theory astonishingly neat and in the lower mid-range level of abstraction. As I will discuss later, decontextualization, while essential, simplifies reality and results in its partial representation.

## Type of Data

What type of data is best for the development of grounded theory? This is an area in which there is some disagreement among grounded theorists. Originally, grounded theory was conducted in a research setting, using both observational and interview data. Strauss notes that such data should be experiential (Strauss, 1987). However, in a recent review article Benoliel (1996) observed the trend away from using observational data, to a reliance on unstructured interviews, which are often not conducted in the research setting.

Let us return to the process criterion. As mentioned, one of the ways that grounded theory is more easily developed, making a process more readily identifiable, is to use data that are continuous over time. Unstructured retrospective interviews, in which participants tell their stories about some event from beginning to end, are a natural foundation on which researchers may identify processes. As participants volunteer their stories, these stories provide data that incrementally build the processes and strategies needed to derive grounded theory.

I have learned the hard way—by struggling to develop grounded theory from interviews that do not have this sequential form or from observational data that were not linked overall—that continuous narrative data are essential. That is, observational data are "snapshots" of a process—field notes record short periods of observations rather than a continuous overview of the process. Such observations may be micro-analytic glimpses—glimpses that do not readily meld to process for developing theory. For instance, observations may be of a particular type of touch, and while the touch itself does provide information and fit into the theoretical scheme, the information does not fit with the developing theory on types of relationships or is not easily understood without the overriding theoretical scheme.

Therefore, researchers should be attentive to the collection of data and the type of data collected for grounded theory analysis. As mentioned earlier, focus group data are not amenable to grounded theory. As conversations about certain topics or opinions, these data contain few stories. Although participants may agree, even nonverbally, these data do not reappear in different forms (as occurs with a saturated data set), and they contain little replication in the sense that is required for saturation. At best, focus group data may be considered disjointed "snapshot" data, poorly suited to grounded theory. These data are not in a continuous form and are not best suited for developing grounded theory.

Let's consider other examples. Interviews may be a collection of short accounts about a topic, and these topics may not be linked to one another—they may be presented as separate, even unrelated, incidents. For instance, one project in which data resisted being molded into grounded theory was one on developing nurse-patient relationships (Morse, 1991). Eventually, data were presented as a list of characteristics, and types of developing relationships were presented in separate lines and not linked elegantly as grounded theory should be. I now understand the underlying problem as being one of competing perspectives. Interaction data (and the methods used by interaction theorists, such as observational method and conversational analysis) do not provide the retrospective, reflective data needed for understanding relationships. Thus, relationship theorists, including grounded theorists, must use retrospective interviews.[2]

Thus the form of data collected demands that certain studies should be analyzed by certain methods. To ignore these criteria that make grounded theory possible neither renders it an easy process nor does it permit the best product to be developed. Data are forced into the form required in order for the researcher to *think* as a grounded theorist.

## Level of Development

The lower to mid-range level of abstraction of grounded theory that so excellently explicates behavioral concepts and behavioral phenomena does not handle broad topics well. For example, with broad topics such as Chronic Illness and the Quality of Life (Strauss, Corbin, Fagerhaugh, et al., 1984) where the focus is less explicit, the context overwhelms and it reads like an ethnographic study.

One strength of grounded theory is its ability to recognize patterns (typologies) of behaviors. While some criticize this approach as removing and simplifying the individual experience, if the theory remains grounded in data, it permits the individual voices to remain. Glaser's (1998) recent admonishment against using recording and transcription, however, limits the ability of the researcher to use the participants' quotations and consequently the ability of the researcher to truly ground the study. Glaser's advice is odd and appears to counter the very principles that Glaser himself advocates.

Keeping grounded theory grounded also limits the level of abstraction. If theory must remain grounded in data, the researcher is restricted—all concepts used must be demonstratedly linked to data.

---

[2]This important point escapes Silverman (1998) who does not appreciate the difference between these methods and their results. Using the inappropriate method to answer a question is not a matter of disciplinary preference and perspective (as Silverman suggests), but a matter of validity and methodological coherence (i.e., using the most appropriate methods to answer the question).

The solution to this problem of developing formal theory from substantive theory begs the question: Because formal theory is decontextualized, is it still grounded? Should it be? Or is it adequate that conceptual linkages "ground" this type of theory?

Processes of decontextualization raise the level of abstraction of a theory by moving it to higher level concepts and, in the process, remove it from the particular context. In this way, the level of generalizability of the theory is increased. The removal of the theory from a particular context eliminates its groundedness—its links to the particular, to the participants, and to the context in which it was created. Linkages to the literature and to established concepts are stronger. Again, is such a theory still grounded theory? I believe formal grounded theory continues to be grounded theory because the structure retains its distinctiveness. Process remains evident and the stages, phases, and core variable remain intact. At the same time, the theory is applicable to many more situations and contexts.

## Use of Induction

The inductive nature of grounded theory was specifically developed to permit creativity and freedom. Glaser (1998) specifically warns the researcher against exploring the literature before commencing data collection, as it may move the researcher too quickly toward completing analysis. There is less chance of forcing or trying to fit the established knowledge. Thus, unique insight into reality and original theory is more likely to be developed from grounded theory.

Such a naïve perspective as working without consulting the literature may be possible for a senior investigator with a vast knowledge of social science theory with many concepts at his or her fingertips and with real theoretical wisdom. However, ignoring the literature is a strategy that is fraught with danger for a new investigator. Literature should not be ignored but rather "bracketed" and used for comparison with emerging categories. Without a theoretical context to draw on, new investigators find themselves rapidly mired in data—the very state that Glaser himself warns against. Or as Brink (1991) noted:

> There are a lot of students out there who cannot think creatively. They are so concrete! They don't have that incredible flight of fantasy that is needed to be a good qualitative researcher. They don't have

the ability to make connections. When they see two pieces of data they say, "Oh, well, I've got two pieces of data! I've got that, and I've got that, and now what do I do?" (p. 300)

New investigators also lack the confidence to trust their own capabilities to create worthwhile research. Being able to compare their findings with others gives them a springboard into the analytic process.

This creative license and the admonishment to ignore the work of others is rapidly producing a rather interesting problem in grounded theory literature. As investigators develop their own set of concept labels in each study, they tend to ignore others' work, refusing to compare their labels with those used by others for the same or very similar concepts. A scramble to identify unique concept labels exists as if a unique name for a concept indicates that a new concept itself has been discovered. Knowledge is becoming redundant, rather than creatively new and exciting. Our literature is becoming noisy and cluttered. Thus we are developing a situation where researchers publish minor studies without linking or situating their studies within the literature pertaining to that topic. The recent trend towards meta-analysis means that researchers must decide, without the benefit of the original data, if two investigators are addressing the same or different concepts. I cannot emphasize strongly enough that the task of associating studies by using the same concept name is the responsibility of the investigator and we must work towards developing more theoretical cohesion among studies.[3] Further, any research under the guise of qualitative meta-analysis is nothing more than "label-smoothing" and does not, as meta-analysis should, develop new models of greater explanatory power.

Stern (1996) provides us with an interesting conceptual framework for women's health in which she uses established theoretical codes from Glaser and Strauss to identify the dimensions for women's health. She links these codes to her data and the work of others. Without the literature such theoretical richness is neither feasible nor possible.

---

[3]This contains the caveat that, in order to preserve induction, these labels must be identified and applied after one's analysis is completed.

## Tolerance of Variation

One of grounded theory's greatest strengths is the challenge it presents to researchers to actively seek variation. While remaining focused on the concept, the grounded theorist's deliberate listing of all data characteristics, comparing and contrasting, coding and verifying, and the purposeful seeking and saturation of negative case sampling ensures rich, dense, comprehensive results. If conducted well, grounded theory is valid, strong, and powerful.

Paradoxically, variation in the sample ensures that bias, while used as a sampling technique, is removed from the final product. The completed theory is presented as a balanced and well-rounded explanatory description of the topic. Note that the active seeking of variation and incorporating it into a model ensures validity. This is one of the major and most important strengths of the method.

## The Soundness of Theory in Grounded Theory

Processes of theoretical construction of grounded theory are unique and systematic processes of conjecture and verification that are the hallmarks of grounded theory methods. It is the incremental development of the theory that is verified with data each step of the way, not the overall verification or theory testing that is conducted after the grounded theory is completed—a point that is confused when discussed by Dey (1999).

Miller and Fredericks (1999) attribute this inductive/deductive process to the processes of discovery and justification used widely in social science, noting that they do not exclude processes of interpretation. Furthermore, as both Glaser and Strauss emphasize causality, the theory produced by grounded theory methods may predict and explain. The result is a very solid and useful theory.

Elsewhere, I have argued that these processes of verification inherent in the construction of theory result in a product that closely resembles reality (Morse, 1997), giving it top marks for validity and representativeness. It remains as theory, however, because of its abstract nature (Morse, 1997).

## The Strengths of Grounded Theory

Excellent grounded theory is an elegant, useful and valid research method and, as such, it has made an important contribution to understanding society's problems. It has been particularly useful for students as its methods and strategies are well described and it keeps students focused, producing research that is manageable for a thesis or dissertation. But if we ask "What makes grounded theory a grounded theory?" most likely we will get the answer that it is a study that is "grounded in the data." Unless, however, there is something unique about "grounded," this is not a comprehensive definition, as all qualitative studies are "grounded in data."

What is grounded? When "appropriate data" were explored above, we found that the form of data played a significant role in the development of grounded theory. The characteristics of these data were continuous over time, experiential, readily conceptualizable, and of adequate variation. Are these unique characteristics? Perhaps. Grounded theory is less concerned with a particular context, cultural perspectives, and world views than ethnography. It is more concerned with how participants create and respond to experiences rather than, as with ethnography, what they think or how they perceive their world.

Nonetheless, "grounded" has something to do with the development of theory from data, and this resulting theory must therefore remain linked to those data. That is, while abstract, the theory must also remain embedded in the context, which is usually presented as the lives of participants. It, therefore, best answers questions that focus on the experiences of participants, documenting their responses through an event. This is probably why grounded theory has played such an important role in nursing. It best answers the concerns and questions that are important to our discipline, such as the illness experience.

Because of the reliance of grounded theory on theoretical form, it is essential for the researcher to understand grounded theory as a method before attempting to do grounded theory. This understanding could be obtained from a mentor, from participating in a seminar or from reading excellent examples of published grounded theory. Strauss is right that grounded theory is a way of thinking

Norris, C. (1990). *What's wrong with postmodernism?: Critical theory and the ends of philosophy.* Baltimore: Johns Hopkins University Press.

Poland, B. D. (1992). Learning to 'walk our talk': The implications of sociological theory for research methodologies in health promotion. *Canadian Journal of Public Health, 83*(2) (Suppl. 1), 31–46.

Richards, T., & Richards, L. (1991). The NUD*IST qualitative data analysis system. *Qualitative Sociology, 14*(4), 307–324.

Sandelowski, M. (1986). The problem of rigor in qualitative research. *Advances in Nursing Science, 8*(3), 27–37.

Sandelowski, M. (1993). Rigor or rigor mortis: The problem of rigor in qualitative research revisited. *Advances in Nursing Science, 16,* 1–8.

Sim, S. (1998). *The Icon critical dictionary of postmodern thought.* London: Icon Books Ltd.

Smith, H. (1995). Postmodernism and the world's religions. In W. T. Anderson (Ed.), *The truth about the truth: De-confusing and re-constructing the postmodern world* (pp. 204–214). New York: Putnam.

Strauss, A. (1993). *Continual permutations of action.* New York: Aldine De Gruyter.

Strauss, A., & Corbin, J. (1990). *Basics of qualitative research: Grounded theory procedures and techniques.* Newbury Park, CA: Sage Publications.

Strauss, A., & Corbin, J. (1994). Grounded theory methodology: An overview. In N. K. Denzin & Y. S. Lincoln (Eds.), *Handbook of qualitative research* (pp. 273–285). Thousand Oaks, CA: Sage Publications.

Thornham, S. (1998). Postmodernism and feminism (or: Repairing our own cars). In S. Sim, *The Icon critical dictionary of postmodern thought* (pp. 41–52). London: Icon Books Ltd.

Wakefield, N. (1990). *Postmodernism: The twilight of the real.* London: Pluto Press.

Wolcott, H. F. (1973). *The man in the principal's office: An ethnography.* New York: Holt, Rhinehart & Winston.

Wuest, J. (1995). Feminist grounded theory: An exploration of the congruency and tension between two traditions in knowledge discovery. *Qualitative Health Research, 5*(1), 125–137.

# CHAPTER 4

# The "How To" of Grounded Theory: Avoiding the Pitfalls

## Rita Sara Schreiber

One of the struggles in teaching and learning grounded theory is that it is difficult to capture fully and in writing the "how to" of the method without sacrificing its more intuitive aspects. Part of the difficulty is that getting a handle on the method involves process learning: you learn it as you do it. The "doing," however, goes much more smoothly and is likely to have better results when the novice is able to work with an experienced mentor who can guide the way. In many graduate programs, mentors are in short supply. Another difficulty is that the only time procedures are not done all at once (rather than linearly, as they are inevitably presented in textbooks) is at the initiation of data collection. Once there are data in hand, the complex, multilayered process of sampling, coding, theorizing, and writing is in full force. It is a challenge, however, to adequately convey the gestalt of this process in words. Thus, the reader should try to visualize the sections of this chapter as forming a layer cake rather than cupcakes; the researcher experiences the whole much more than the pieces.

A few authors have actually attempted to describe the grounded theory research process in some detail, most notably Glaser (1978),

Strauss (1987), and Strauss and Corbin (1990, 1998), however these works are limited in light of developments in the method (see, for example, MacDonald, this volume). Melia (1996) and others (J. Morse, personal communication, August 30, 1996) have criticized Strauss and Corbin (1990, 1998) in particular as having reduced the rich complexity described in Glaser and Strauss (1967) to a linear and formulaic recipe. Although some of the criticisms, such as coding minute pieces of data, have been addressed in the recent edition, some of the book's limitations remain. For example, Strauss and Corbin (1998) have kept the discussion of such procedures as the "flip-flop technique," in which "a concept is 'turned inside out' . . . to obtain a different perspective . . . " (p. 94), although other research-ers have seen it as a forced and unhelpful comparison (Glaser, 1992). In my experience, Glaser (1978) continues as the best single resource for the novice researcher, however, not all students find it fully accessible.

Having outlined in advance the challenge of describing in writing how to do grounded theory, my purpose in writing this chapter is to do just that. I have structured the chapter around certain problematics that, in my experience, can lead to difficulty for the learner of grounded theory. Although I recognize the challenge of trying to convey to a novice the gestalt of grounded theory through the linear reading/writing process, I hope, by focusing on these problematic areas, to help smooth the learning process. The wise novice grounded theorist, however, will not mistake my construction of the process for Truth but will use it as a place to begin, as well as a basis for comparison with the writing of others. What I will discuss is my understanding of how I do a grounded theory study.

## THE METHOD

Glaser and Strauss originally published their work on grounded theory in 1967, and since that time, the method has been further refined and explicated by numerous others, notably Williams (1989), Glaser (1978, 1992), Strauss, (1987), Chenitz and Swanson (1986), Stern (1980, 1985, 1994), Hutchinson (1986), Strauss and Corbin (1990, 1994, 1998), Wuest (1995), and Wuerst & Merritt-Gray (chap-ter 8, this volume). Its roots are in factor analysis (P. Stern, personal communication, May 12, 1994), pragmatism, and symbolic interactionism. As an exploratory method of research, grounded theory does not begin from a position of an existing theory and pre-defined concepts. Rather, as the researcher collects, codes, and analyzes data (which might be journals, group or individual interviews, field notes, books, videos, and/or other narrative forms), concepts and properties emerge (Glaser & Strauss, 1967).

Writers sometimes refer to grounded theory as the constant comparative method because coded data are constantly compared with other data and concepts at each level of theory development. At each stage of analysis, the researcher generates hypotheses or hunches about relationships between and among categories that are tested against the data. The researcher continues to compare emerging conceptualizations, which result from testing these hypotheses, against the data until core categories and a theory of behavior are distilled and understanding of human experience from the perspective of the participant is advanced. However, there is more involved in doing grounded theory than constant comparison.

I have found grounded theory to be useful when we want to learn how people manage their lives in the context of existing or potential health challenges and as such, is admirably suited to nursing inquiry. What is key in this process is learning the ways that people understand and deal with what has happened to them through time and in changing circumstances. Grounded theory is also useful for research in areas that have not previously been studied, where there are major gaps in our understanding, and where a new perspective might be beneficial.

## REVIEW OF THE LITERATURE

Students who have read either *Discovery* or *Theoretical Sensitivity* often are mystified by the originators' advice to omit the usual literature review in favor of direct investigation of the phenomenon of concern. Rather than being swayed by the great minds of the past, Glaser and Strauss admonished grounded theorists to formulate their own interpretations, based on participants' understandings of what was going on. In keeping with the modernist focus on the experience of the common (hu)man and concurrent rejection of research driven by *a priori* theory, this notion represented a shift away from the domination of positivist ideals in social science and nursing research. Thus, in a perfect grounded theory world, students might have been advised to limit prior reading to an exploration of grounded theory as a methodology with its epistemological and ontological roots, and prior grounded theory studies.

There are, however, methodological reasons for conducting a literature review. Glaser (1978, 1998) and Strauss and Corbin (1998) suggest that reading related and unrelated technical and popular literature is a good way to expand one's ideas about the matters under study and to help promote theoretical sensitivity (see below). In addition, the researcher brings to the study an existing background familiarity, gained through reading of professional or popular literature. Few researchers approach a topic without past experience and a continued interest in it. (The wise doctoral student bears this in mind when selecting a dissertation topic with which to live intimately for several years.) The researcher, however, cannot "unlearn" what is already known, therefore, the risk of conducting a literature review is that the researcher might superimpose his or her preconceived ideas onto the data. By conducting a formal literature review, the researcher can fully explicate many of her or his existing conceptualizations and sensitizing concepts (see below) of the phenomenon of study and subject them to the challenge of ongoing comparison with data. Thus, the researcher uses constant comparison to scrutinize the literature for its fit with emerging concepts and theory to better ensure the rigor of the findings.

More pragmatically, the current expectations of academic research and funding agencies suggest that plunging into field research without delving into the relevant literature would be folly. At the very least, researchers need to be aware of previous writing about the topic in order to develop a proposal aimed at adding something new. Having this knowledge, the researcher can also gain an appreciation for the magnitude of the problem, and thus, the importance of conducting the proposed study. Often, reviewing the academic literature is of limited use, since it rarely is focused on the problem of a given population as identified by that population. Nevertheless, the researcher who is seeking funding must demonstrate an understanding of the "state of the science" regarding the phenomenon of study in order for agency evaluators to be confident that their money would be well-spent. Thus, in today's world a literature review is usually a necessary first step in beginning any research project, including a grounded theory.

## SENSITIZING CONCEPTS

As suggested above, a sensitizing concept is an idea or understanding the researcher already has in her or his head about the phenomenon of study. A sensitizing concept may also be one identified from the research, popular, or practice literature that, in the researcher's mind, seems salient. The researcher may or may not be aware of the ideas and preconceived notions she or he holds and should make efforts to uncover and challenge them. The idea of identifying sensitizing concepts can be traced back to Blumer (1969/86) who suggested that concepts identified from prior sources must be carefully scrutinized and only brought into the study if support is found in the data. Glaser (1978) and Glaser and Strauss (1967) concur with this view. For example, in my studies of women and depression, I identified key concepts such as learned helplessness or attachment/loss as having been plausibly linked with depression in women. Because of this, I was alert to anything in the data that might reinforce or refute these concepts. I found, however, that these concepts could account for only a very small portion of the data.

Identification of sensitizing concepts should not be an excuse for superimposing one's favorite theory onto the data, however, and the researcher must remain vigilant against this possibility. For example, Milliken (1998) initiated a study of parental caregivers of adults with schizophrenia using loss and grief as sensitizing concepts. Although she found ample evidence of these concepts in the data, her rigorous scholarship allowed the data to override her preconception, to learn that the role of loss and grief was not as central as she had anticipated. In Milliken's study, the central issue (and basic social process) was "Redefining Parental Identity" in which participants changed how they understood themselves and their identity as parents as a result of having an adult child with schizophrenia.

Thus, although there may be merit for a researcher to approach a study in a *tabula rasa* fashion, it is not likely to be realistic or feasible to do so. To quote Dey (1993), "There is a difference between an open mind and an empty head. . . . The issue is not whether to use existing knowledge, but how" (p. 63). What is needed is for the researcher to recognize her or his own assumptions and beliefs, make them explicit, and use grounded theory techniques to work beyond them throughout the analysis.

To do this, the researcher may explicate in writing her or his pre-existing notions and carefully scrutinize them against the data. A research seminar or study group can be very helpful in this process, and colleagues who are not as enmeshed with the subject matter can often provide fresh insights to challenge you when you get stuck on an idea or concept. Likewise, when group members have heard you discuss the same (or similar) conceptualizations repeatedly, they can provide confirmation that the data support your findings, even though you are doubting yourself. Thus, by constantly comparing sensitizing concepts with data, the researcher can move beyond preconceptions toward the construction of a fully developed theory that is rooted in and explains the data.

## THEORETICAL SENSITIVITY

Theoretical sensitivity is another way the researcher guards against potential biases that can be a threat to the rigor of the study. Theoretical sensitivity is the ability of the researcher to think inductively and move from the particular (data) to the general or abstract, that is, to build theory from observations of specifics. This process begins when the first data are in hand, as the researcher immediately examines the data from both the particular and the abstract levels, asking "what's going on here?" The researcher must be able to imagine, and test against data, a variety of explanations (theories) of what the data say. The personal background of the researcher is the filter of salience through which data are sieved, and each researcher is more or less open to theoretical possibilities contained within a data set; however, each must cultivate this ability. Development and refinement of theoretical sensitivity requires vigilance and practice.

Theoretical sensitivity helps curb the potential bias from the researcher's background experiences and diminishes the risk of compromising the study through premature closure in favor of the researcher's pet theory. One technique for promoting theoretical sensitivity is to memo one's pet theories and set them aside for later comparison against the data. This is not the same as bracketing, as used in other interpretive traditions, because grounded theorists recognize that the researcher and her or his experience cannot be removed from the process. Some would argue that personal experience with the phenomenon of study is vital to the analysis process. Thus, the researcher explicates his or her background knowledge, not to isolate it from the study, but with the specific intention of bringing it into the analysis to see if the data are supportive or not.

To cultivate theoretical sensitivity, the researcher must recognize and constantly challenge her or his personal theories and biases against the data. This constant comparison allows for the emergence of theory that is truly grounded in data. For example, at the time Stern was doing her dissertation research on how stepfather families handled matters of child discipline, most writers advised couples to agree on the rules prior to marrying (Kiely, 1976). However, Stern's theoretical sensitivity allowed consideration of a variety of possible theoretical explanations for what was happening in the data so that she could discover that family rules of discipline were largely implicit and unspoken. Further, family members did not discover the rules until after they broke them (Stern, 1977).

The researcher can improve her or his theoretical sensitivity by attending to all possible explanations for what one sees in the data, particularly in light of negative cases (data that disconfirm or refute an emerging hypothesis). This involves inductive logic, moving from the specific observation to the theoretical level. For example, a class-room exercise I like to use is presenting an observation (for instance, "Nurses working in your facility have noticed that bedridden aboriginal elders do not seem to suffer skin breakdown as much as other elderly patients") and asking the group to brainstorm as many possible explanations (theories) for this as they can. The range of explanatory theories offered is always diverse and creative and includes everything from physiology to social behavior (family members turn elders more frequently than nurses turn other patients). I use this exercise to demonstrate both the range of theories that might emerge from a single observation and the usefulness of discussing one's emerging ideas in a group.

Discussing with others the categories and emerging theory, and examining how it all fits (or not) together, can assist the researcher in keeping perspective and not getting lost in the endlessly ruminative process of analysis. This also helps keep the analysis grounded in the data and not in the researcher's imagination where it too easily slips. The challenge for the researcher is to be open to the theories that are in the data, but not to get lost either in the data's minutiae or in theorizing. The researcher must also listen when others observe that the categories seem forced and be prepared to step back from the analysis and take a fresh look. Outside readers, colleagues, and participants can be very helpful here.

## THE PROBLEM

Grounded theorists begin with an assumption that participants share a problematic situation, which they (participants) may or may not articulate. Even though the researcher tries to approach the study "with as few predetermined ideas as possible" (Glaser, 1978, p. 3), she or he cannot unlearn what is already known. Thus, even the act of selecting something to study imposes a pre-existing conceptual structure onto the phenomenon. The researcher has already identified what she or he thinks the problem is and begins the study from that perspective. However, the first goal of the researcher is to understand the shared basic social problem from the participants' perspective. Their understanding of the problem must be revealed so that the grounded theory will reflect what participants do to resolve it. Novice researchers sometimes omit this important first step, and this can lead to difficulty when trying to explicate how participants resolve the problem. Since the grounded theorist's ultimate goal is to learn how participants resolve or ameliorate the shared problem, it is vital to first learn what the problem really is.

For example, MacDonald (1998) conducted a study of implementation of a drug and alcohol prevention program that involved the introduction of prevention workers into the school system. Based on her reading of the literature, she was interested in learning whether the program would be implemented as it was intended. However, neither MacDonald nor the designers of the prevention program anticipated that prevention workers could not begin implementation until they had established themselves as credible and welcome in the schools. Thus, the basic problem discovered in the field was how prevention workers established themselves in their schools so that they could begin to implement the program. MacDonald's resulting theory reflected the complex balancing of political and personal intents revolving around the prevention worker role, and it was far richer and more explanatory than if MacDonald had forged ahead without uncovering the real basic social problem.

## PARTICIPANTS AND SAMPLE SIZE

The grounded theorist faces recruitment issues similar to those in other research studies based on interview data, and he or she is bound by ethical considerations of self-selection, confidentiality, no risk to treatment (if recruiting in a treatment setting), and so forth (Holloway & Wheeler, 1995; Morse, 1998; Robley, 1995). Depending on the topic, participants may find the interview process to be emotional, yet often helpful (Draucker, 1999). In the case of interviewing on sensitive topics (such as sexual abuse or depression) or with vulnerable people, a procedure for prompt referral and support should always be established in the event that an untoward outcome should arise from the interview.

An exact determination of the size of the population for a study cannot be established *a priori* (Morse, 1991, 2000; Sandelowski, 1995). It is important to remember that the units of analysis are not predetermined and are not known until the data are in hand. The units of theoretical analysis are not the individual participants themselves, but may be incidents, stories, examples, and so forth. For example, in one study of oncology nurses and do-not-resuscitate (DNR) decision making, the units of analysis were discrete patient/family scenarios. Each nurse interviewed contributed several scenarios which resulted in more than 100 units of analysis (Jezewski & Finnell, 1998). Much depends on the scope and complexity of the study, the number and range of potential participants (how large and homogeneous is the group?), the design of the study (repeat interviews or single? participant observation?), the quality of the data, how reflective (and talkative) the informants are, and other parameters such as the realities of graduate studies. If the researcher is lucky and finds a number of reflective and articulate participants, the number of interviews needed might be less. Similarly, participant observation in the field can add volumes of data relatively quickly. In general, the more widespread and varied the data, the larger the data set must be to reach theoretical saturation; however, the researcher must keep in mind that variation is needed for theory development.

## THEORETICAL SAMPLING

Grounded theorists use theoretical sampling, the process of simultaneously collecting, coding, and analyzing data to generate theory. Theoretical sampling is a complex, changing process that shifts as the categories develop and the theory emerges. Because of this, the researcher can only plan in advance the initial sampling for data collection. This contrasts with positivist or "normal" science (Kuhn, 1970) in which the sampling procedure is designed in advance and adhered to rigorously. Instead, the sampling process is entirely controlled by the emerging theory (Glaser & Strauss, 1967). A good grounded theorist will seek out more than one data source to provide a wider perspective on the phenomenon of study. For example, a researcher studying depression and treatment might want to interview knowledgeable patients, nurses, psychiatrists, and psychologists. She or he might also want to examine hospital records so that many, varied perspectives are revealed. Each of these data sources would provide valuable, yet different, information about depression and treatment. By seeking different perspectives on a topic, the researcher is challenged to develop explanations for the variation in the data and to unify them at a more abstract level into a theory.

As categories emerge, the researcher targets certain groups or subgroups for data collection, first to test and refine the emerging categories, and then to elaborate and saturate them. For example, when doing early sampling for a study on depression, I discovered an over-representation of nurses and other care providers. To correct this, I sought informants in other occupations (for example, outside the caring professions) to ensure sufficient diversity to test the emerging conceptualizations.

As the researcher develops hunches about what is going on in the data, she or he might want to explore various circumstances under which an event does or does not happen, which might mean asking more specific questions or seeking out particular types of informants. For example, a researcher studying how people of sexual minority orientation manage life at a university (S. Vilches, personal communication) found visibility in the classroom to be an issue for everyone. However, further questioning people of sexual minority orientation[1] revealed context-specific strategies for managing visibility. Many opportunities arose, such as classroom discussions of family structure, in which a student chose (or chose not) to speak up and raise awareness of sexual minority issues. Speaking up depended on whether: (a) the person felt there was a chance she or he would actually be heard, and (b) she or he felt it was important *in the particular situation* to ensure the atmosphere was safe for people of sexual minority orientation. If these two conditions were not met, the student kept silent and remained on the margins. In this case, the researcher had some notion of what might be going on and selected key informants to ask specific questions to test her hypotheses.

The researcher usually continues theoretical sampling throughout the study. Often, while writing the theory, it is necessary for her or him to keep sampling in key areas to help fill in the categories or flesh out the connections between them.

## DATA COLLECTION

In grounded theory everything is data. This means that, when the grocery store clerk learns that the researcher is studying house fires and she begins to talk about when her house burned down, the researcher listens and learns. Depending on the quality of information relayed, the researcher may give it more or less weight than other data, but this woman has shared data that also go into the pot with the rest. The researcher may even want to ask if the woman is

---

[1]The project included both those who identified themselves as people of sexual minority orientation and those who did not.

willing to be interviewed. A TV show about people's experiences with house fires is also good data, as are diaries, magazine articles, and other first-hand accounts. Depending on the study scope and on what is emerging from the data, the researcher may also examine fire department records or other documents. It is all data, and good grounded theories are built on a variety of data sources and perspectives on the topic, but the choice of data source is determined and directed by the emerging theory.

Most nurse researchers rely on formal and informal interviews as core sources of data in their studies. My experience suggests that the best (and most likely) site to conduct interviews usually is the participant's home or in a private office, however, my experience might not be typical. I would not interview street people, for example, in either of those settings. It is important that the interview be conducted in a quiet, private place where the participant will feel comfortable and where interruptions can be kept to a minimum.

Not all grounded theorists agree that interview taping is absolutely necessary (see Morse, chapter 1, this volume and Stern & Covan, chapter 2, this volume), so long as the researcher takes detailed, legible notes that she or he can read later (Glaser, 1998). I am reluctant to make a habit of conducting untaped interviews because I have found taking detailed notes to be distracting, and making legible notes impossible. Further, I have found considerable important detail in transcribed interviews that I would likely have lost through note-taking. Regardless of whether or not tape recording is used, it is imperative to memo or record one's impressions of the interview as soon as possible afterward, or important details will be lost. May (1994) has suggested keeping the tape recorder on until after the researcher and participant have said their good-byes, and the researcher is in the car, so that the nuggets of information that so often emerge on the doorstep are not lost.

The researcher continues collecting data until saturation is reached. Saturation, often called "theoretical redundancy," occurs when the categories and theory are fully explicated and no new information about the core processes is forthcoming from ongoing data collection (Strauss & Corbin, 1998). This may not happen until late in the final write-up because it is in committing the theory to the page that the researcher may discover gaps in the data. When this happens, the researcher must identify the best sources of data to answer the questions that will fill these gaps. Sometimes graduate committees, especially at the master's level, limit the scope of a study for purposes of completing a program. In such circumstances, the novice grounded theorist develops a theory that may not have all of the categories fully saturated. There are no "hard and fast" rules related to theoretical sampling for saturation. Instead, the researcher must keep in mind the purpose of the data collection and the relevance to the emerging theory, and not get sidetracked (which is too easy to do).

## USE OF AN INTERVIEW GUIDE

It is often advisable for beginning researchers to develop either a draft interview schedule or at least a list of topics to be covered, which provides novices with a quick reference in case of nervousness or forgetting. As a very nervous novice researcher, I was comforted to hear Katharyn May (1994) state that many of her earliest interviews were embarrassing for her to read later, and that some of them should probably have been discarded. Nonetheless, with a bit of experience, it becomes easier to ignore the interview schedule and follow the trail of the interview as the participant tells it. This approach is preferable, as the primary job of the researcher is to discover the participants' understandings of how they resolve the problem under study. Imposing the interviewer's structure will affect the quality of data received. Then, once the participant has told the full story in his or her own words and probe questions ("anything else?") have been asked repeatedly, the researcher can briefly look at the interview schedule and check whether anything has been missed. This approach prevents the researcher from foreclosing on the participant's reality in favor of her or his own anticipated agenda.

Several tricks of the trade may be useful. Two key questions to help finish an interview are: (a) What advice would you have for someone experiencing (the phenomenon of study)? and (b) Is there anything else I should know about (the phenomenon of study) that I didn't ask? These two questions prompt the participant to reflect and often lead to fruitful data. Another useful technique, once the interview is nearly completed, is to pose direct questions about conceptual relationships, based on the literature, or (more likely) on emerging concepts or hunches. For example, one might say something like, "Others have told me (or, "The literature suggests . . . ") that . . . Has this been your experience?" This allows the person to say "No, not really" or to validate the hunch and elaborate on what it has meant for her or him.

This latter technique illustrates how the interview schedule changes over the course of the process. The researcher draws such key questions from the analysis to promote theory development. For example, toward the end of a study on women's experience with treatment and depression (Schreiber & Hartrick, in press), it became clear to members of the research team that, although many women told personal stories of psycho-social challenges and traumatic experiences, their understanding of what would help them get better was medication. After hearing this several times, we began asking women directly if they could explain the connection between what they said led to their depression and what they felt was needed to make things better. This was important for us, because we were trying to elucidate the role of treatment in recovery from depression. This type of questioning allowed us to develop a theory to describe how women adopted a biomedical explanation to explain their depression and manage its stigma.

Thus, the grounded theorist changes the interview questions over the course of the study, moving from the general ("Tell me about your experience with X") to the specific ("How is X situation like Y for you?"). As the researcher gains skill in developing key questions from the data and conducts more interviews, she or he can move away from an interview guide to follow the data. After each interview, most researchers find it helpful to write memos about impressions, ideas, and so forth arising from the interview. Researchers also find it useful to make specific notes of areas to cover or specific questions to ask in future data collection.

## ANALYSIS OF DATA

### Coding

Through conceptual coding the researcher transforms raw data into theory. By coding data and comparing the codes with the data, the

undertake data collection and analysis. The application of analysis of difference to grounded theory has the potential to improve the accuracy and legitimacy of the research process and findings. Recognizing socioeconomic, ethnic, sexual, cultural, and other differences between researcher and participant makes explicit the researcher's place in the process and findings, as well as leading to a better understanding of the basic social problem, that is, the processes through which participants make meaning in their lives. As such, an analysis of difference contributes to the development of substantive and formal theories that inform our comprehension of participant's lives.

## QUESTIONS AND FINAL THOUGHTS

When I began this research project (Mallory, 1998), I struggled with a number of methodological issues. In this chapter I have attempted to answer some of the questions generated by that process. As much as I would like to end the whole thing with a tidy conclusion, I do not think such a thing exists in grounded theory. Instead I am left with a sense of how complicated and problematic an analysis of difference may be. For example, could accounting for difference be interpreted as forcing data into preconceived categories that have meaning only to the researcher? Also, how much sensitization prior to data collection is necessary in order to anticipate difference, and could this sensitization blind the researcher to characteristics, values, and beliefs that they hold in common with participants? Under what circumstances should inquiry into difference be undertaken, and when would a study benefit from such analysis? Would an analysis of difference detract from the collection of other, more relevant, data? In addition, there are practical considerations: how might the researcher approach the documentation and reporting of difference within a grounded theory study, and are we asking too much of the participant in commenting on difference?

Plainly, there is much room for discussion on the appropriateness and application of analysis of difference to grounded theory. I am convinced, however, that those of us who have chosen to use grounded theory need to consider carefully how differences may separate us from those from whom we would learn. Without the recognition and examination of differences along ethnic, cultural, economic, social, and sexual lines, we remain limited as instruments of research. Whatever we aspire to in our research, at the very least it is understanding, and, perhaps for some, an analysis of difference will expand our understanding.

# REFERENCES

Anderson, J. M. (1991). Reflexivity in fieldwork: Toward a feminist episte-mology. *IMAGE, 23*(2), 145–148.

Bunting, S. M. (1997). Applying a feminist analysis model to selected nurs-ing studies of women with HIV. *Issues in Mental Health Nursing, 18,* 523–537.

Bunting, S., & Campbell, J. C. (1994). Through a feminist lens: A model to guide nursing research. In P. L. Chinn (Ed.), *Advances in methods of inquiry for nursing* (pp. 75–87). Gaithersburg, MD: Aspen.

Campbell, J. C., & Bunting, S. (1991). Voices and paradigms: Perspectives on critical and feminist theory in nursing. *Advances in Nursing Science, 13,* 1–15.

Glaser, B. G. (1978). *Theoretical sensitivity.* Mill Valley, CA: The Sociology Press.

Glaser, B. G., & Strauss, A. L. (1967). *The discovery of grounded theory: Strategies for qualitative research.* New York: Aldine Publishing.

Guba, E. C. (1990). The alternative paradigm dialog. In E. G. Guba (Ed.), *The paradigm dialog* (pp. 17–27). Thousand Oaks, CA: Sage Publications.

Hall, J. A., & Stevens, P. E. (1991). Rigor in feminist research. *Advances in Nursing Science, 13*(3), 16–29.

Mallory, C. (1998). Women on the outside: The threat of HIV and margin-alized women. (Doctoral dissertation, Indiana University, 1998). *Disser-tation Abstracts International 59-09,* 4729.

Maynard, M. (1994). Methods, practice and epistemology: The debate about feminism and research. In M. Maynard & J. Purvis (Eds.), *Researching women's lives from a feminist perspective* (pp. 10–26). London: Taylor and Francis.

Robrecht, L. C. (1995). Grounded theory: Evolving methods. *Qualitative Health Research, 5*(2), 169–177.

Stanley, L., & Wise, S. (1993). *Breaking out again: Feminist ontology and epistemology.* London: Routledge.

Stern, P. N. (1994). Eroding grounded theory. In J. Morse (Ed.), *Critical issues in qualitative research methods* (pp. 212–223). Thousand Oaks, CA: Sage Publishing.

Stern, P. N., Allen, L. M., & Moxley, P. A. (1984). Qualitative research: The nurse as grounded theorist. *Health Care for Women International, 5*, 371–385.

Stern, P. N., & Pyles, S. H. (1986). Using grounded theory methodology to study women's culturally based decisions about health. In P. N. Stern (Ed.), *Women, health and culture* (pp. 1–24). Washington: Hemisphere Publishing Corporation.

Wuest, J. (1995). Feminist grounded theory: An exploration of the congruency and tensions between two traditions in knowledge discovery. *Qualitative Health Research, 5*(1), 125–137.

# CHAPTER 6

# The Grounded Theory Club, or Who Needs an Expert Mentor?

## Rita Sara Schreiber

Grounded theorists, particularly those who learned their trade from either Glaser and Strauss or from their direct disciples, have long espoused the view that one cannot learn to do grounded theory without a mentor. Having learned grounded theory in this way, I, too, endorsed this notion that the student of grounded theory would necessarily be lost without the guidance of a far wiser, more experienced teacher in the method to guide and assist the learner. Yet recent experiences have caused me to question this belief and consider wider conceptualizations of mentorship in this context.

This chapter represents my thoughts on the process of learning grounded theory and the nature of mentorship in that process. I wrote this because I have yet to find very much written on how to begin to learn grounded theory. In this chapter, I will briefly touch on the original teaching of grounded theory to graduate students at UCSF, identifying key strategies foundational to student learning. I will also outline some developments within the field that could profoundly impact the teaching, learning, and practice of grounded theory. Following this, I will propose an alternative model for teaching and learning grounded theory that has recently emerged, the Grounded Theory Club (GTC), and reflect on the role of expert mentoring in learning grounded theory.

## EARLY TEACHING AND LEARNING

When Glaser and Strauss were first developing the method, the primary venue for teaching research methodology was a sequence of five graduate quarters of seminars entitled "The Discovery of Social Reality," held at the University of California at San Francisco. Both Glaser and Strauss conducted seminars within the sequence at various times. This was an exciting time to be a graduate student at UCSF, and the seminar was highly prized by those who attended. (Stern and Covan, who were there at the time, have discussed this period of history in chapter 2, this volume.) What is important about this time is that an enriched atmosphere was created in which variation in perspective added to understanding and helped novice researchers wrestle with their data and tease out the core concepts of their studies.

In this atmosphere, students could gain an appreciation for the "magic" that is part of the process of doing grounded theory research (Glaser, 1978; May, 1994; Morse, 1991). As Barney Glaser is fond of pointing out, the core concept is probably buried in the first interview, but the researcher cannot yet see it. It is only once the researcher has collected, analyzed, and wallowed in much more data, and enjoyed some respite as well, that the magic of "discovering" the grounded theory can happen (Glaser, 1978).

Central to this teaching/learning experience is the notion that there are expert mentors who could guide students in gaining an understanding of the methodological considerations that applied to their own particular studies. This mentorship is viewed by many grounded theorists as the only way in which one can truly learn grounded theory, or at least learn it properly (Stern, 1994; May, 1994; May & Hutchinson, 1994). Mentorship styles have varied. Some, like Glaser or Strauss, took on the role of expert at whose feet novice researchers might learn the method. Such expert mentorship could be enacted in various ways, depending on the personality of the mentor. The power and influence, however, remain firmly with the expert. Such an expert mentor might work closely with students, helping them code interviews and pointing out issues and questions to attend to in later interviews and memos. Some expert mentors might also identify a likely core concept of the study, helping the student to focus more closely on what is salient. In this way, expert grounded theory mentors seem to have taken a high-support approach to guiding novice researchers. In spite of differences in mentoring styles which might suit different learners, mentorship has always been an important feature in learning grounded theory.

Without such mentorship, however, students have been left to wander on their own, trying to use a method they have never seen enacted and trying to make sense of their data with no glimpses of how this might happen. This has often been the case for the poor graduate student wanting to do a grounded theory study but finding himself or herself in a department without a qualitative researcher, much less a grounded theorist. Without appropriate mentorship, many novice grounded theorists were forced to do the best they could. Sometimes the results were quite satisfactory (Milliken, 1996), however, most of us are familiar with the wide range of poor scholarship that some authors thought was grounded theory (May & Hutchinson, 1994; Stern, 1994). There can be no doubt that having a good mentor can only improve the overall quality of research that is published under the guise of grounded theory.

## THE GROUNDED THEORY *OEUVRE*

For a long time, there was very little in the way of practical guidance that a novice grounded theorist might find in the literature. There was *Discovery* (Glaser & Stern, 1967), of course, plus *Theoretical Sensitivity* (Glaser, 1978), and two articles by Stern (1980, 1985), but these were not particularly directive in terms of providing a "how to" that would assist the novice. *Discovery* provided a philosophical argument, largely in positivist terminology, for why grounded theory could be a valid and reliable research methodology. The work of Glaser (1978) was more directly applicable and contained helpful sections on coding, memoing, and theory development, however, the reader was still left to his or her own imagination to figure out how the theoretical discussions of these methodological issues could apply to his or her particular study data. It was not until the appearance of Strauss'

*Qualitative Analysis for Social Scientists* in 1987, which walked the reader through careful examples of research data, that a novice grounded theorist could begin to get a picture of how to pull it together and what it all meant. Indeed, a careful reading of these three sources can provide an excellent theoretical understanding of what grounded theory is all about, but the researcher is still left to develop what it might look like for one's own particular research interests.

Since 1986, there has been a proliferation of literature on the methodology, including Strauss and Corbin (1990a & b, 1998), Glaser's response to Strauss and Corbin (Glaser, 1992), Hutchinson (1986), Chenitz and Swanson (1986), and others (Annells, 1996; Glaser, 1994, 1998; May, 1996; Melia, 1996; Strauss & Corbin, 1994). Strauss and Corbin's 1990 attempt to make the grounded theory method transparent has been widely read (1990a). It has also been widely criticized by some grounded theorists who view it as a cookbook in which the method has been reduced to a simple step-by-step recipe. It has been criticized in a more personal manner by Glaser who, in addition to seeing it as reductionist (and therefore not the "true" grounded theory), appears to have had some personal ax to grind. This interchange has long been discussed and debated, with various respected scholars firmly and convincingly supporting one side or another. (See MacDonald, chapter 7, this volume, for a new perspective on this apparent schism.) The substantive debate and criticism following publication of Strauss and Corbin (1990a) led to a newer edition in 1998 in which many of the criticisms of the earlier version were addressed.

We have found that the apparent schism between Glaser and Strauss has led some graduate committees to try to steer students away from grounded theory, in the fear that the student will become enmeshed in an incomprehensible and nonproductive debate. We have learned, however, that when the issues are explicated, some of the fears of our academic colleagues have begun to dissipate. To be sure, it is not entirely clear that grounded theorists outside of nursing consider this debate to be of any substance. In fact, from a teaching and learning perspective, the apparent argument between Glaser and Strauss has proven to be a real boon to grounded theory, as it has attracted attention and provoked a flurry of excited debate, both in print (Annells, 1996; Melia, 1996; Stern, 1994) and in corridors. This has, in turn, stimulated a spurt of new development of the methodology as people are challenged to reconsider their assumptions and beliefs about research.

Of equal importance is the fact that this Glaser-Strauss controversy created widespread public discourse about the method as well as its epistemology, ontology, and application. This discussion is accessible to anyone who takes the time to read the literature on grounded theory carefully and critically. This means that even the unfortunate graduate student stranded in a department full of post-positivists can sift through the discourse and begin to make his or her own sense of what grounded theory is in a much more informed way than was possible even 10 years ago. Further, if she or he has a colleague in a similar position, they can share resources, thoughts, ideas, criticisms, and challenges to push each other further in their own development as researchers. In this way, the presence of a body of literature on the method and the various perspectives from which grounded theory has been viewed has provided a valuable resource that was missing when many of us were trying to learn it.

In addition, the dialogue that is now underway provides a variety of perspectives that the novice researcher must address. Without addressing them, the student cannot understand what grounded theory means for her or him. This situation puts much more responsibility at the feet of the learner than was previously necessary or even possible. Instead of either being handed the method by a mentor or being left to guess the method, the learner now must sort through all the philosophical and practical considerations and arguments to discover what she or he understands as grounded theory methodology and how it might be used to study the particular phenomenon of interest. It is from these humble beginnings of recognizing that we are all learners on this stage that the Grounded Theory Club emerged.

## THE GROUNDED THEORY CLUB

The Grounded Theory Club (GTC) emerged when a handful of faculty new to the University of Victoria School of Nursing realized that we were all using or had used grounded theory in our graduate work. A fourth sessional instructor was considering grounded theory as he developed his doctoral proposal. Thus, it seemed like a good idea to get together occasionally and talk about grounded theory issues. An early consideration was that we were an island of symbolic interactionists within an ocean of phenomenologists, and we had a vague sense that we could support each other. We knew we were lucky in not having to work in a post-positivist environment, but we wanted to ensure the survival of an interactionist perspective within the prevalent discourse.

It did not take long before graduate students and others began to hear about the group and wanted to attend. This led to the eventual current composition and format of the GTC. The group meets approximately every two weeks for two hours and is open to anyone interested in grounded theory. In this way, members range from those who have done one or more (funded) grounded theory studies through those who are just trying to figure out the difference between the various interpretive/constructivist methods and identify what would best fit their own research interests. This variation in background enables us to have lively, ongoing consideration and reconsideration of anything related to the method and its application.

In true grounded theory fashion, what has emerged was not envisioned at the outset. From my own perspective, it seems that we have developed three main scholarly purposes:

1. Teaching/learning
2. Consideration of emerging issues/development of the method
3. Mutual mentorship

## Teaching/Learning

The core of the GTC is teaching and learning of grounded theory. Located as we are within the culture of the Faculty of Human and Social Development, we conceptualize teaching and learning from an emancipatory perspective (Friere, 1974; Allen, 1990). From this perspective, the expertise of the teacher is not in the content to be learned but in the process of how to learn, and the most effective learning is transformational in nature (Mezirow, 1991). Learning is created through the process of engagement with the material through discussion and dialogue so that the learner is transformed through the process. In this way, we are all co-learners in the GTC, and this becomes evident at each meeting as we discuss our own creation of knowledge. This means that there are no experts in the GTC, although some members have more experience than others. Members of the GTC bring to meetings whatever issues each would like to see addressed. An agenda is created and we consider each issue in turn. A typical agenda might be:

- Tina's data
- Sampling
- Brainstorming/finding Jane's theory
- The nature of theory in grounded theory

Frequently, one or more issues must be shelved for a future meeting, or, if all are equally important, a special meeting will be scheduled. In this way, we have, thus far, been able to make sufficient time to address fully whatever methodological issues arise.

Having the range of experience within the group has enabled us to think through why we do what we do when we are involved with a study. For example, students considering whether or not to use grounded theory or phenomenology have provided us the opportunity to explore the philosophical underpinnings of both methods so that they could decide which approach better suited their research interests. Consideration of the ontology and epistemology of the two methods helped them identify how a study would be different depending on which direction was selected, but it also allowed each of us the opportunity to explicate our own natural biases.

Often at meetings, members writing dissertations or theses have shared drafts of grounded theory schematics with the group for discussion. This has led to discussion and questions about the emerging theory and helped clarify the final product. This also provided the opportunity for everyone to get involved with various ways that other literature might enlighten the discussion section of the dissertation. For example, one member described her early findings in a study of the process of parenting an adult child with schizophrenia. The category under discussion concerned the way in which parents, frustrated by their inability to effect change in the care their own children received, turned to social action and began working for improved care for all people with schizophrenia. This led to discussion of a paper by Covan (1995), remembered from a conference in which adults living far from their elderly parents tended to informally "adopt" another elderly person to care for, in a symbolic enaction of caring for a loved one without directly providing that care. The open discussion also provided some guidance for others' work and the applicability (or not) of the concept of symbolic or substituted caring and arguments that might be pursued for their own research.

Another teaching/learning approach that has recently emerged has been in the classroom. Instead of inviting a token grounded theorist to guest lecture in graduate or undergraduate courses, instructors have been inviting the GTC to attend classes and hold a mock meeting. In these circumstances, as many members as possible attend, and we form a circle-within-the-circle of the classroom. In most instances, someone will give a brief overview of what grounded theory is and an example of a grounded theory. If the class is in a graduate course, a more specific topic, such as sampling or data analysis, might be the focus. After this, the floor is open for very informal discussion of issues that arise from the group. Members of the GTC come prepared with questions to pose in case they are needed, however, this has never been the case. More often than not, the students themselves have burning methodological issues, as they have their own research concerns.

One of the earliest questions that arises is whether or not it is appropriate (or necessary) to do a literature review to do a grounded theory study. As novice researchers, graduate students have often expressed feeling caught between knowing they must write a proposal and having read in *Discovery* that "the truth is out there somewhere" rather than in the literature. This has always led to a discussion of the practical realities of graduate school as well as understanding sensitizing concepts. Within the context, a discussion of the applicability and feasibility of bracketing and its relationship to grounded theory often arises. This usually helps students who are having difficulty making sense of the disparate perspectives to recognize their own needs as researchers.

The benefits of this approach to introducing students to grounded theory is that they can see it as a living, breathing methodology. They can be introduced to some of the issues and perspectives that are currently part of the discourse among grounded theorists without being overwhelmed or discouraged from trying it. In fact, the GTC has gained members through contact with students in this way, as they have come to realize that their confusion is normal.

## Consideration of Emerging Issues/Development of the Method

One of the early benefits that emerged from the GTC meetings has been ongoing discussion of emerging issues within the field. This began, as might be expected, with discussion of the Glaser-Strauss debate, as the more experienced members considered themselves at that point to be Glaserian grounded theorists. Early discussions justified this position. More than one person, however, had a need to explore whether or not grounded theory as a method would accommodate incorporation of a critical theory perspective, and this led to a review of the origins of the method. It was through this review, largely led by Marjorie MacDonald, that members began to realize that perhaps the Glaser-Strauss debate was a red herring founded on very little substance and that what we thought the masters' positions were was, to some degree, illusion. This has enabled us to explicate what each has written and to more clearly delineate our own perspectives on grounded theory. It has also allowed us to understand the areas of congruency between grounded theory and critical social theory in their philosophical origins and thus, contribute, in some small way, to the development of the method.

At GTC meetings, we have discussed other developments and their applicability to grounded theory. In one recent meeting, we discussed the relative merits of using computer applications to manage data. Currently, three members of the group use NUD*IST, while a third uses Atlas-ti to code and manage their data. In other meetings, we have considered the applicability of post-modernist thought to grounded theory methodology, and we have come to some surprising understandings (see MacDonald & Schreiber, chapter 3, this volume). On several occasions, we have taken up the issue of whether or not grounded theory is wedded to symbolic interactionism, and whether such a marriage is one of convenience or of true kinship (see Milliken & Schreiber, chapter 9, this volume). At the same time, the dialogue about the compatibility of grounded theory with a critical perspective has also become ongoing, particularly as new graduate students come with their own needs to "make a difference" for/with participants. In this way, we are working toward a fuller understanding of the method within the larger methodological discourse.

## Mutual Mentorship

The original purpose of the GTC was to provide each of us on the faculty with support to keep going with our various research projects. This is ongoing, and most welcome. We had no way of anticipating, however, how important this would become for the student members of the group, as they often feel lost in trying to design their own graduate research projects. When they are able to bring their questions, and to learn that their questions are important to ask, it is easier for them to decide whether they want to try grounded theory or not. Those who do not do this at least understand more clearly why they prefer another method, while those who do use grounded theory have a venue to bring forth their issues, concerns, and triumphs as they work through the process. This has been rewarding for all of us.

As members reach various stages of their data collection and analysis, they present their findings, at whatever stage, to the group and seek assistance in sorting things out. This is in keeping with Glaser's (1978) suggestion that the process is enriched by other perspectives, and by gaining some distance from time to time from the data. At a recent GTC meeting, two members presented their findings. One, a student, was in the middle of data collection and was beginning to formulate ideas of what might be hiding in the data. Members helped her by raising questions, suggesting possible contingencies, and providing ideas for areas to pursue in further interviews. For example, the student, who was studying student activism in high schools, noticed a difference between students at two different schools. Possible explanations for this included different school cultures, different student organizations, different individuals within the groups, and so forth, giving direction for areas in which the data could be saturated further. In contrast, another member, who was struggling to finish her dissertation, was supported by members to stop wallowing in the data and "just write." Several practical suggestions for this were offered, including inserting "insert juicy quote here" in the text instead of being tempted to search for the best quote, which could be done later. In these ways, both practical and personal support have become integral to the GTC, as we have all been co-learners in creating the process.

## DO YOU NEED AN EXPERT MENTOR?

As interest in interpretivist/constructivist research has flourished, awareness of the complexity of the ontological and epistemological issues surrounding methodology decisions has grown. This has promoted the growth and evolution of various methods, including grounded theory, as different views of the philosophical issues emerge. Indeed, different observers of grounded theory have described it as situated within a variety of traditions, including postpositivism (Denzin & Lincoln, 1994; Guba & Lincoln, 1994), interpretivism (Annells, 1996; Stern, 1994; Strauss & Corbin, 1994), and constructivism (Annells, 1996). The field is getting more complex and difficult to navigate without help finding the signposts.

Occasionally, someone will have the fortitude and drive to tease through the literature on his or her own and figure it out, but he or she will often report feeling lost and unsure even after having completed the project. This is especially the case with a first project, and the results are often of poor quality (Susan Noakes, personal communication). It is not likely that most people can learn to do grounded theory without at least some guidance and support. Why would anyone want to do something the hard way when help is available? But what does that guidance and support look like?

Much depends on how we view grounded theory itself. If we view grounded theory as a fully developed method of inquiry, then we do, indeed, need to learn its True Enactment from an expert so that we can ensure the proper use of it. In this case, there is little need to continue discussing it. However, if we can understand grounded theory as evolving, changing, and growing, then we, as co-learners, can promote both our own understanding and the development of the method through sharing our ideas in the general discourse. This is the perspective taken at the GTC, and I believe such collegial approaches can help ensure that we are not eroding grounded theory

(Stern, 1994) but rather building on it, ensuring its rigor, and explicating its usefulness.

Nonetheless, the chance to work with an originator of grounded theory, or with a direct descendant, still exists. The relatively easy availability, through phone, fax, and e-mail, of such leaders as Stern, Benoliel, and May, among others, presents a precious opportunity for those who would seek such guidance. In my experience, most methodologists are only too happy to speak with learners who call them seeking assistance, even if the person is a complete stranger. Yet, I have always been surprised at how few people, struggling alone with an idea, will pick up a phone and directly ask a few questions of someone who might be able to provide some clarification. The availability of these senior grounded theorists will not last forever.

What withstands through time, however, is what can be found in the literature: the writings of the masters, their disciples, and any other interpreters. Anyone with a commitment to understanding grounded theory can read what has been written and make meaning of it in his or her own way. It is through this interpretive process *about* grounded theory that new ideas are raised and the methodology is developed. Although some writers may feel that what they have written stands on its own and requires no interpretation, the reality is that, each time we read something, we interpret its meaning. In this way, the writings are cast and re-cast in different epistemological contexts so that they gain new, or enhanced, meanings in time.

This message was brought home to me through a multimedia piece of art I happen to own. At the time I acquired it, the artist told me how she had come to create the piece in response to her child's sorrow and rage at the artist going away for a week. For years, whenever people commented on the "unusual" piece (doubtless a euphemism), I explained that it had to do with the feelings of the person "left behind." When I re-encountered the artist and told this to her, her response was, "Well, that's what I created. But it's your painting now, so it can mean whatever you make of it." The message is that we put our ideas out into the fray of the discourse, but how it is received, both immediately and in time, is subject for interpretation and reinterpretation.

All this is a circular approach to answering the original question: Do you need a mentor to learn grounded theory? Consultation with an expert can be a priceless and important experience for learners of grounded theory. Having the opportunity to show one's work to a more experienced expert and receive feedback is invaluable in developing both confidence and knowledge of the research tradition. The learnings that we can gain from direct contact with experts should be considered an important source of data in figuring out what grounded theory is. It is not to be mistaken, however, for received wisdom or Truth, which can stifle learning and growth. This is where I believe mentorship has sometimes become synonymous with capital "m" method, as in Methodolotry.

We can, however, reconceptualize mentorship from the hierarchical origins of the term and its early enactment, including within the grounded theory tradition, to a more egalitarian understanding of the concept. If mentors are seen as co-learners with particular areas of expertise, then mentorship can promote an emancipated approach to learning grounded theory. Each of us has something to teach and something to learn about grounded theory, even if it is only by raising old or dumb questions. In this way, peer mentorship, such as practiced in the GTC, is available to everyone who wants it and who is truly committed to engaging in a learning process. Such mentorship benefits both students and faculty, and the existence of research interest groups such as the GTC has been identified as a characteristic of top-ranked schools of nursing (Pollock, 1986).

My personal truth is that it is not the mentor *per se* that makes the difference. I believe that anyone engaged in scholarly inquiry who is committed to understanding what grounded theory is all about does not need an expert to tell him or her. What he or she needs is to make use of all the resources available, including the growing body of literature, consulting with colleagues, and consulting with the experts. Engaging in the dialogue to discover what grounded theory is and how it works, the learner will recognize his or her own understanding as he or she triangulates the disparate data sources. In doing so, the learning of grounded theory will ultimately emerge for each who seeks this knowledge.

## REFERENCES

Allen, D. G. (1990). Critical social theory and nursing education. In N. Greenleaf (Ed.), *Curriculum revolution: Redefining the student teacher relationship* (pp. 67–86). New York: NLN.

Annells, M. (1996). Grounded theory method: Philosophical perspectives, paradigms of inquiry, and postmodernism. *Qualitative Health Research, 6*(3), 379–393.

Chenitz, W. C., & Swanson, J. M. (1986). *From practice to grounded theory.* Mill Valley, CA: Addison-Wesley Press.

Covan, E. K. (1995, October). Caregiving near and far: A discussion of transference and burnout. Paper presented at the Biennial North American Congress on Women's Health Issues, Galveston, TX.

Denzin, N. K., & Lincoln, Y. S. (1994). Introduction: Entering the field of qualitative research. In N. K. Denzin & Y. S. Lincoln (Eds.), *Handbook of qualitative research* (pp. 1–18). Thousand Oaks, CA: Sage.

Friere, P. (1974). *Pedagogy of the oppressed.* New York: Seabury Press.

Glaser, B. G. (1978). *Theoretical sensitivity.* Mill Valley, CA: Sociology Press.

Glaser, B. G. (1992). *Basics of grounded theory analysis.* Mill Valley, CA: Sociology Press.

Glaser, B. G. (1994). *More grounded theory methodology: A reader.* Mill Valley, CA: Sociology Press.

Glaser, B. G. (1998). *Doing grounded theory: Issues and discussions.* Mill Valley, CA: Sociology Press.

Glaser, B., & Strauss, A. (1967). *The discovery of grounded theory.* Chicago: Aldine.

Guba, E. G., & Lincoln, Y. S. (1994). Competing paradigms in qualitative research. In N. K. Denzin & Y. S. Lincoln (Eds.), *Handbook of qualitative research* (pp. 105–117). Thousand Oaks, CA: Sage.

Hutchinson, S. (1986). Grounded theory, In P. Munhall & C. Oiler (Eds.), *Nursing research: A qualitative perspective* (pp. 111–130). New York: National League for Nursing.

Hutchinson, S. A. (1993). Grounded theory: The method. In P. L. Munhall & C. O. Boyd (Eds.), *Nursing research: A qualitative perspective* (pp. 180–213). New York: National League for Nursing Press.

May, K. A. (1994). Abstract knowing: The case for magic in method. In J. M. Morse (Ed.), *Critical issues in qualitative research methods* (pp. 10–21). Thousand Oaks, CA: Sage.

May, K. A. (1996). Diffusion, dilution, or distillation? The case of grounded theory method. *Qualitative Health Research, 6*(3), 309–311.

May, K. A., & Hutchinson, S. A. (1994, June). Grounded theory: The method. Symposium presented at the 3rd International Qualitative Health Research Conference, Hershey, PA.

Melia, K. M. (1996). Rediscovering Glaser. *Qualitative Health Research, 6*(3), 368–378.

Mezirow, J. (1991). *Transformative dimensions of adult learning.* San Francisco: Jossey-Bass.

Milliken, P. J. (1996). Seeking validation: Hypothyroidism and the chronic illness trajectory. *Qualitative Health Research, 6*(2), 202–224.

Morse, J. M. (1991). Qualitative nursing research: A free-for-all? In J. M. Morse (Ed.), *Qualitative nursing research* (pp. 14–22). Thousand Oaks, CA: Sage.

Pollock, S. E. (1986). Top ranked schools of nursing: Network of scholars. *Image, 18*(2), 58.

Stern, P. N. (1980). Grounded theory methodology: Its uses and processes. *Image, 12*(1), 20–23.

Stern, P. N. (1985). Using grounded theory in nursing research. In M. M. Leininger (Ed.), *Qualitative research methods in nursing* (pp. 149–160). New York: Grune & Stratton.

Stern, P. N. (1994). Eroding grounded theory. In J. M. Morse (Ed.), *Critical issues in qualitative research methods* (pp. 212–223). Thousand Oaks, CA: Sage.

Strauss, A. (1987) *Qualitative analysis for social scientists.* Cambridge: Cambridge University Press.

Strauss, A., & Corbin, J. (1990a). *Basics of qualitative research: Grounded theory procedures and techniques.* Newbury Park, CA: Sage.

Strauss, A., & Corbin, J. (1990b). Grounded theory research: Procedures, canons, and evaluative criteria. *Qualitative Sociology, 13*, 3–21.

Strauss, A., & Corbin, J. (1994). Grounded theory methodology: An overview. In N. Denzin & Y. Lincoln (Eds.), *Handbook of qualitative research* (pp. 273–285). Thousand Oaks, CA: Sage.

Strauss, A., & Corbin, J. (1998). *Basics of qualitative research: Grounded theory procedures and techniques* (Second edition). Newbury Park, CA: Sage.

# CHAPTER 7

# Finding a Critical Perspective in Grounded Theory

## Marjorie MacDonald

> In the social sciences there is only interpretation. Nothing speaks for itself.
>
> —Norman Denzin, 1994

> The most creative thinking occurs at the meeting places of the disciplines.
> At the centre of any tradition, it is easy to become blind to alternatives.
> At the edges, where the lines are blurred, it is easier to imagine that the world might be different.
>
> —Mary Catherine Bateson, 1989

In the wake of the Ottawa Charter for Health Promotion (World Health Organization, 1986), nurses have been trying increasingly to articulate the meaning of health promotion for their research and practice (Lowenberg, 1995; Novak, 1988; Rush, 1997). As a nurse educator who is interested in community health promotion, I have been fairly clear about the implications of health promotion theory for my own teaching and practice. As a researcher, however, I found myself wondering about relevant methodologies for studying health promotion, given the potential conflict between assumptions inherent in some qualitative research methodologies and in the philosophical underpinnings of health promotion. Because I saw a need for the development of health promotion theory in nursing, I was drawn to grounded theory as a research methodology. However, given my commitment to the Ottawa Charter version of health promotion, with its inherently critical perspective, I was concerned about whether grounded theory as an interpretive methodology would be appropriate for my own research.

Although others have argued that grounded theory can be integrated with a feminist methodology (e.g., Wuest, 1995; current volume), which is one of a number of critical theories (Stevens, 1989), no one has argued the case clearly enough for my needs that grounded theory can address specific charges that arise from explicitly critical perspectives, including the socio-ecological perspective of health promotion. At the very least, the origins and epistemology of grounded theory raised initial questions for me about its relevance in a field, such as health promotion, that is simultaneously concerned with both macro- and micro-social issues. My preliminary reading on Symbolic Interactionism (SI) and grounded theory suggested that they were focused primarily on the micro-social world of situated interaction. I was most concerned about charges that SI and, by extension, grounded theory did not address social structural issues (Denzin, 1992; Reynolds, 1993). If this was true, I reasoned, then its relevance for studying health promotion might be limited.

My explorations, however, led me to conclude that grounded theory is an appropriate methodology for studying health promotion for two main reasons. First, the originators of grounded theory have always been concerned not only with social psychological processes but also with social structural processes and the structural conditions that influence those processes, although these have not been emphasized in most of the published grounded theories by nurses. Second, grounded theory's relevance for health promotion research is related to the consistency among key concepts of SI, the socio-ecological perspective in health promotion, and critical social theory. These will be discussed later in this chapter.

In this chapter, I describe my own scholarly journey to determine the relevance of grounded theory as a methodology for studying health promotion phenomena. This was a rather convoluted journey that took me across a vast terrain. I began by exploring the philosophical and conceptual foundations of grounded theory to identify potential sources of conflict and compatibility with the socio-ecological perspective of health promotion. As I got into this literature, it became clear to me that the answer to my question might be different depending on which version of grounded theory (if there really is more than one) I was considering. This led me to an analysis of the so-called schism between Glaser and Strauss (and their respective followers). From there, I followed the implications of this analysis for the way grounded theory could be used in health promotion research. Before I describe my journey, however, I will begin by clarifying what I mean when I use the term "health promotion."

## HEALTH PROMOTION

My understanding of health promotion and its historical development has been articulated elsewhere (MacDonald, in press), but a brief overview of what I mean when I use the term will help to situate the later discussion. Maben and Macleod Clark (1995) argue that health promotion, particularly in nursing, is a contested concept and that the meaning varies from one person to the next. Many people see it as being synonymous with health education and having a focus on changing lifestyle behavior (Kulbok, Baldwin, Cox, & Duffy, 1997; Pender, 1987, 1996). This individualist view of health promotion has been entrenched in health policy in some countries, including the United States and Great Britain, but it is not consistent with the more collectivist perspective articulated in the World Health Organization's Ottawa Charter which defined health promotion as "the process of enabling people to increase control over, and to improve, their health" (World Health Organization, 1986, p. 1). The Ottawa Charter identified the importance of social factors in determining health by naming the fundamental prerequisites to health: peace, shelter, a stable ecosystem, sustainable resources, social justice, and equity. Writers of the Charter also proposed that the major health promotion strategies are building healthy public policy, creating supportive environments, strengthening community action, developing personal skills, and reorienting health services. Thus, although a health promotion perspective does not preclude an individual focus at the micro social level, the emphasis is on understanding and taking collective action on the social and environmental influences on health at a macro social level. Elsewhere (MacDonald, in press), I have described the parallels between a health promotion perspective as per the Ottawa Charter, and an emerging critical social perspective in nursing (Butterfield, 1990; Kendall, 1992; Stevens, 1989; Stevens & Hall, 1992).

Since the Ottawa Charter was released in 1986, the socio-ecological perspective on health promotion has continued to evolve. Stokols (1992) suggests that ecology, which had its earliest roots in biology, is about the interrelations between organisms and their environments. It has evolved in several disciplines into a general framework for understanding the nature of people's transactions with their environments. Social ecology is concerned with social, institutional, and cultural contexts of people-environment relations. Thus, an important assumption in this perspective is that people-environment interactions are characterized by cycles of mutual influence. The assumption of mutual influence is important to remember when I later discuss SI and its relevance to health promotion. It is this assumption that removes health promotion from the realm of a purely structural perspective that would place it at odds with an interpretive research methodology such as grounded theory.

## PHILOSOPHICAL AND THEORETICAL FOUNDATIONS OF GROUNDED THEORY

An in-depth review of SI is beyond the scope of this chapter. I will, therefore, provide only a brief overview with specific attention to ideas that are relevant to the central thesis of this paper. Symbolic interactionism, as a theoretical perspective, was derived from the philosophy of pragmatism, articulated at the turn of the century by Charles Pierce, William James, and John Dewey (Münch, 1994). The sociological perspective that emerged from pragmatism placed particular emphasis on the symbolic nature of social life, which was studied initially from the micro-social perspective of human actors involved in symbolically defining their situations, their selves, and their roles in social interaction. Thus, symbolic interactionists view human beings as active participants and creators of the world in which they live.

Many social theorists saw SI as being in distinct opposition to the classical European sociological perspective which was concerned with macro-social analyses of societal structures (e.g., economy, polity, culture) as the primary determinants of human action (Münch, 1994). Thus, symbolic interactionism emerged as a reaction to the dominance of structural-functionalist perspectives in sociology. For this reason, and because of its emphasis on personal meaning-making in shaping human behavior, symbolic interactionism has been interpreted by many as being unconcerned with the influence of social and structural conditions on human action. This has been called the "astructural bias" (Reynolds, 1993).

The most important contributor to the development of what came to be known as SI was George Herbert Mead who synthesized pragmatism with Darwin's theory of evolution (and thus its links to ecology) and behaviorism. Mead conceptualized the development of self and society as an interaction between the person and his or her natural environment. Herbert Blumer, a sociologist of the Chicago School, further developed Mead's SI into a distinct sociological paradigm and formally articulated the methodological position associated with this perspective (Blumer, 1969). In fact, Blumer officially coined the term "symbolic interactionism" in a 1937 article (cited in Blumer, 1969). Blumer identified three basic premises of SI: (a) human beings act toward things on the basis of the meanings that these things have for them; (b) the meaning of objects derives from social interaction; and (c) meaning is arrived at through an interpretive process.

The starting point for analysis in SI is the notion of "human society as action" (Blumer, 1969). Society is not a structure that exists independently of people's actions and interactions. Rather, human society consists of people engaging in action. Group life (i.e., society) presupposes individual and collective interaction. Human society consists of people in association who interact predominantly on a symbolic level. In contrast to the structural-functional perspective, in which behavior is seen as a product of the factors influencing it, symbolic interactionists see the human actor, not as a responding organism but as an acting organism who constructs his or her own action on the basis of the interpretations made in the course of social and self-interactions.

In Blumer's view, meanings themselves are important, not the apparent structures or systems created by collective, repetitive action. Just because meanings are unquestioned, unconscious, and reflected in prevailing norms, values, and beliefs does not mean that they are not "subtended by a process of social interaction, a process that is necessary not only for their change, but equally well for their retention in a fixed form" (Blumer, 1969, p. 19). According to Blumer, it is the social process of group life that creates and upholds the rules, not the rules that create and uphold group life. It is this principle, in particular, that is challenged by the more structural approaches. In health promotion rhetoric, the importance of social and environmental factors in producing and reproducing health and health behavior has been central. How and whether such rhetoric flies in the face of SI is open to debate and will be taken up below.

## CRITICISMS OF SYMBOLIC INTERACTIONISM AND GROUNDED THEORY

Denzin (1992) has summarized the major criticisms of symbolic interactionism that have emerged over the years. In addition to the charge of an astructural bias, several authors have criticized SI for being ahistorical, apolitical, acultural, overly rational, and non-emotional. It is important to note that many of these criticisms emerged from within the SI tradition itself, thereby leading to concerted efforts by many interactionists to address these issues themselves. Nonetheless, debate has continued over a number of years, within and outside the SI tradition, in relation to these criticisms (Alexander, Giesen, Münch, & Smelser, 1987; Huber, 1974; Layder, 1982, 1989a, 1989b; Meltzer & Herman, 1990; Prendergast & Knotternerus, 1993; Reynolds, 1993; Vaughn & Reynolds, 1968).

The most damaging criticism of SI from both a sociological and a health promotion perspective is that it suffers from an astructural bias. This issue has also been characterized as the "macro-micro debate" or as the case of "structure versus agency." Those charging SI as having an astructural bias believe that symbolic interactionists are not able to deal with macro-structural issues, that is, they fail to deal with social organization and social structure as important influences on human action. Put another way, symbolic interactionists are accused of not adequately recognizing the objective constraints on social action that stem from economic, social, and cultural circumstances, or from race, gender, and ethnic discrimination. Critics have also argued that symbolic interactionists ignore how the interpreted meanings of individuals are channelled by society's dominant institutions.

In response to these criticisms, Denzin (1992) reviewed the large body of interactionist writing that "addresses head on the questions of social structure, social organization, power, the economy, capitalism, history, class structure, race and gender" (p. 59) and concluded that many interactionists have not neglected social structure, especially since the mid-1970s. Some critics (e.g., Meltzer & Herman, 1990) also concluded that symbolic interactionists have contributed to the understanding of social structural influences on human interaction and therefore argue that the notion of the astructural bias as a defining feature of SI should be reconsidered. In fact, the Society for the Study of Symbolic Interaction, which was founded in 1975, considered the solution of the astructural bias to be one of its main purposes (Prendergast & Knotternerus, 1993).

Many of the criticisms of SI are based on the "canonical" texts, especially by Mead and Blumer. Symbolic interactionism, however, has a much more variegated and richly textured history of which critics may be unaware. Denzin (1992) defines six moments of symbolic interactionist theory: (a) the canon (1890–1932), (b) empirical/theoretical period (1933–1950), (c) transition/new texts (1951–1962), (d) criticism/ferment (1962–1970), (e) ethnography (1971–1980), and (f) diversity/new theory (1981–1990). The transition/new text period radically altered the perspective, and Strauss' 1959 work, *Mirrors and Masks*, contributed to this. The criticism/ferment period was a phase of internal critique by symbolic interactionists during which several challenges to the basic premises of SI were published and which led to theoretical and empirical efforts to address the criticisms. Denzin includes Habermas (1987) in the diversity/new theory period, and it is clear that elements of Habermas' critical theory have their roots in symbolic interactionism (Maxwell, 1997) and pragmatism (Antonio, 1989; Shalin, 1992).

Concerns about an astructural bias in SI have been translated into criticisms directed against grounded theory methodology (Layder, 1982, 1989a, 1989b). Perhaps criticism is not an entirely accurate descriptor. Layder finds much to commend in the methodology of grounded theory, but he argues that it needs to attend to the macro-micro problem if it is to move forward. Layder acknowledges the grounded theory premise that there are problems with research beginning from a formalized explanatory framework that proceeds to explain "results" in terms of that framework. Thus, Layder believes that grounded theory "holds out the promise of a healthy theoretical anarchy" (Layder, 1989a, p. 53). At the same time, he believes that this promise is unfulfilled because many grounded theorists hold inflexibly to their methodological positions and thus exclude them-selves from the important wider debates in the philosophy of so-cial science.

Grounded theory has an enduring respect for the empirical world and the perspectives of the people being studied. But, because theory is linked so closely to empirical "reality," Layder argues that grounded theory is limited to what can be observed or recorded about human behavior and the action/interaction among people. As such, it has the potential for a conservative bias and may serve to support and maintain the status quo (Layder, 1989a). The entire thrust of grounded theory is tied to the empirical world as it appears to our senses (Layder, 1989a). This is evident in Glaser's (1992) unyielding trust in the ability of the data to "speak for itself" and to reveal all that is relevant to the analyst who is both persistent and has faith. He believes that if structural conditions are important to the manage-ment of a basic social process, these will emerge in the data. This belief has been criticized by feminists (e.g., Stanley & Wise, 1983) as advancing a form of inductive positivism, especially with the emphasis placed on the "emergence" of categories and the "discovery" of theory (Henwood & Pidgeon, 1995).

In challenging the grounded theory notion that categories related to structural conditions will emerge naturally, Layder (1989a) argues that many aspects of social institutions or power relations are not visible or detectable with a methodology that stays focused on observ-able behavior and peoples' perspectives within particular settings. Although behavior and personal meaning may be accessible through empirical observation, this is not always true of structural phenomena, which may not have observable indicators in the empirical data. Power is not usually addressed in grounded theory, yet power is embedded in our systems of stratification, in gender and ethnic relations, and in other structural phenomena that Layder argues exist separately from people's acknowledgment or understanding of them and which have "real" effects on people's lives. These arguments reflect basic assumptions of critical theories (Stevens, 1989), including feminist perspectives.

There are good reasons why critics have charged both SI and grounded theory with an astructural bias. In reviewing two important texts, one by Glaser and Strauss (1967) and one by Blumer (1969), it is difficult not to make the judgment that grounded theory does indeed ignore issues of power, culture, social organization, economics, gender, and other structural influences on human action. For example, Glaser and Strauss (1967) say "Why not take the data and develop from them a theory that fits and works instead of wasting time and good men in an attempt to fit a theory based on 'reified' ideas of culture and social structure?" (p. 262). Blumer (1969) also emphasized that the phenomena of concern to symbolic interactionists are "acting units" rather than the "structures" and "systems" that are found in orthodox sociological approaches. When Layder wrote his critique of grounded theory, however, he did not have access to Strauss' later writing (Strauss, 1993) which appears to be an attempt to address many of these concerns.

Layder is correct when he says that grounded theory emphasizes the importance of processes of interaction and the way in which individuals and collectives play a part in constructing their social environment. One might argue that this interactionist perspective is indeed the strength of grounded theory and wherein lies one of its major contributions. Certainly, understanding an issue or concern from the perspective of those affected by it is a basic tenet of both health promotion and various critical perspectives, especially feminism, thus strengthening the position that grounded theory is an appropriate methodology for examining health promotion phenomena.

Most grounded theorists have used the methodology for the purpose of micro-level analyses. This is particularly true in nursing. Hutchinson (1986), says that the purpose of grounded theory is to discover and conceptualize the essence of complex interactional processes. This understanding permits the development of relevant nursing interventions. She goes on to note that most of the grounded theories in nursing focus on micro analyses of social processes and do not address the relevant macro analyses of social structural processes. This is likely because much of nursing is concerned with individual care and face-to-face interaction and most nursing theories have an individualistic focus. One exception is community and public health nursing in which population and community level issues are important and the social-structural influences on health are critical foci of emerging community nursing practice (Stevens & Hall, 1992; Kendall, 1992).

Nursing, however, and other health disciplines, are moving away from an individualist perspective, particularly with the increasing emphasis on the importance of health promotion practice (Clarke & Mass, 1998; Duncan, 1996; Williams, 1989). More and more, health promotion practitioners are becoming concerned with societal level concerns and the way social structures and institutions influence health and health behavior. They recognize that these structural factors may be more important in affecting the health of communities and populations (versus individuals) than most health care services (World Health Organization, 1986).

The solution, according to Layder, is that grounded theory must attend to macro phenomena without compromising its concern with the micro world of situated interaction. Macro and micro realms are, after all, mutually interdependent. This interdependence must be captured in the procedures of the method. An amended grounded theory, he argues, would therefore focus on the linkages that bind macro and micro phenomena together. Layder proposes a "research map" to support his "revised" grounded theory position. This map attempts to address the problem of bringing the macro and micro analyses closer together. He attempts to convey the interwoven nature of different levels and dimensions of social "reality." These levels are the self, situated activity, setting, context, and history. Self includes biographical experiences and social involvements. Situated activity involves the dynamics of face-to-face interaction. Setting is comprised of the immediate features of the social environment (e.g., schools, family, neighborhood, community). Context involves macro social forms (e.g., class, gender, ethnic relations). History is woven in at each of the levels, as is power. These elements operate in two

**TABLE 7.1**  *(continued)*

| Analytic Category | Glaser (1992) | Strauss & Corbin (1990) |
|---|---|---|
| Techniques for Enhancing Theoretical Sensitivity (TS) | • Personal characteristics of the researcher necessary for TS but training in theoretical codes is also important to be aware of them and sensitive to their emergence.<br>• TS defined as the ability to generate concepts.<br>• Opposes Strauss and Corbin's strategies for enhancing TS.<br>• Says these are totally unnecessary if one sticks to the original way of doing grounded theory as outlined in *Discovery* and *Theoretical Sensitivity*. | • Personal characteristics of researcher are important for TS, i.e., insight, awareness of subtleties, capacity to identify relevance.<br>• TS comes from personal & professional experience, the literature, and the analytic experience itself.<br>• Insight & understanding increases in interaction with data.<br>• State that there is difficulty in striking a balance between one's own knowledge and holding onto the "reality of the phenomenon."<br>• Suggest concrete strategies to deal with this problem: questioning, detailed analysis of word or phrase, flip flop technique, systematic comparison of phenomena (perhaps unrelated to data), far out comparisons, and waving the red flag. |

*(continued)*

**TABLE 7.1** *(continued)*

| Analytic Category | Glaser (1992) | Strauss & Corbin (1990) |
|---|---|---|
| Coding Types | • Initially, 3 types of coding: open coding, theoretical coding and constant comparative coding. Later added selective coding.<br><br>1. Open coding—initial stage of constant comparative analysis, before delimiting to the core category<br>2. Theoretical coding—a property of coding that yields the conceptual relationship between categories and their properties<br>3. Constant Comparative Coding—coding incidents for their categories and properties, and the theoretical codes that connect them<br>4. Selective coding—to cease open coding and to delimit coding to only those variables that relate to the core variable in sufficiently significant ways to be used in a parsimonious theory. | • 3 types of coding: open coding, axial coding and selective coding.<br><br>1. Open coding—the process of breaking down, examining, comparing, conceptualizing and categorizing data<br>2. Axial coding—data put back together in new ways after coding, by making connections between categories using a coding paradigm (causal conditions, phenomenon, context, intervening conditions, action/interaction strategies, consequences)<br>3. Selective coding—process of selecting one category (core), systematically relating it to other categories, validating relationships, and fitting in categories that need refinement. |

**TABLE 7.1** *(continued)*

| Analytic Category | Glaser (1992) | Strauss & Corbin (1990) |
|---|---|---|
| | • The basic questions to ask of the data while coding are: What is this a study of? What category or property of a category does this incident indicate? Any other questions pre-conceive the data and force them into categories that do not fit.<br>• Glaser charges that Strauss's emphasis on the coding paradigm and dimensions concentrates on only two of the 18 coding families described in *Theoretical Sensitivity* will result in something other than grounded theory. It forces the data to fit "pet" codes rather than to allow the data to dictate the coding family it belongs to. | • Two analytic procedures are central to coding: asking questions and making comparisons. Asking questions opens up the data (e.g., who, what, where, when, why) and leads to theoretical sampling.<br>• Questions will differ according to coding type and are generative of the analysis.<br>• Emphasize the dimensions of each category. |

*(continued)*

**TABLE 7.1** (*continued*)

| Analytic Category | Glaser (1992) | Strauss & Corbin (1990) |
|---|---|---|
| Open Coding | • Open coding begins with no concepts and ends when a core category is determined.<br>• Glaser charges Strauss with "overconceptualizing" the data and that the procedures Strauss uses proliferates codes unnecessarily.<br>• Glaser says open coding does not involve as much fracturing of an incident as Strauss suggests because this generates an unwieldy number of codes, because Strauss asks preconceived questions, rather than just the neutral questions of GT.<br>• Strauss' questioning process in open coding represents the "irretrievable, irresistible shift from the fundamental point of GT."<br>• Glaser says Strauss focuses on "dimensionalizing" the categories and properties, but dimensions are only one of the 18 coding families proposed in *Theoretical Sensitivity*. Dimensions may not be relevant in the data. | • Open coding does not necessarily end when a core category is identified. Rather, it is identified during selective coding.<br>• During open coding the data are broken down into discrete parts, closely examined, compared for similarities and differences and questions are asked.<br>• Strauss maintains that each time an instance of a category occurs in the data, it is possible to locate it along a dimensional continuum. |

**TABLE 7.1** (*continued*)

| Analytic Category | Glaser (1992) | Strauss & Corbin (1990) |
|---|---|---|
| Axial Coding | • Glaser maintains that axial coding is entirely unnecessary in GT. "We do not link categories using the paradigm model. The theorist simply codes for categories and properties and lets whatever theoretical codes emerge where they may." <br><br>• Strauss' paradigm model is the same as the 6C coding family described in *Theoretical Sensitivity*. It is only one of 18 coding families. Limiting the coding to the 6C's preconceives the data and will not allow a grounded theory to emerge. <br><br>• Glaser says Strauss has abandoned the concept of theoretical coding as presented in *Theoretical Sensitivity*. <br><br>• Charges that Strauss presents two definitions of "context" which are in conflict. <br><br>• Glaser argues that the relationships between the categories are self-evident and will simply emerge. | • Axial coding is a set of procedures whereby data are put back together in new ways after open coding by making connections between categories. This is done by means of a coding paradigm involving the following categories: causal conditions, phenomenon, context, intervening conditions, action/interaction, consequences. <br><br>• Strauss and Corbin do not talk specifically about theoretical coding, but the ideas seem to be inherent in their description of axial coding, although they are primarily restricted to the paradigm categories. In Strauss and Corbin (1994) they discuss the importance of theoretical coding. <br><br>• In doing axial coding, the researcher asks questions about the relationships between the categories then goes back to the data to verify those relationships. <br><br>• Sometimes it is necessary to track down relationships if you come across something in the data that appears to be related to something else. |

*(continued)*

**TABLE 7.1** *(continued)*

| Analytic Category | Glaser (1992) | Strauss & Corbin (1990) |
|---|---|---|
| Selective Coding | • Selective coding means to cease open coding and to delimit coding to those variables that relate to the core variable in sufficiently significant ways to be used in a parsimonious theory.<br><br>• In GT, selective coding occurs only after the analyst has found the core category.<br><br>• Claims that integration of the theory (which occurs at the stage of selective coding) is not difficult; it just happens in sorting the theoretical codes. " . . . it just happens, because the world is integrated and we are discovering the world, not creating it."<br><br>• Claims, in contrast to Strauss, that discovering the core category is automatic and easy.<br><br>• Says that Strauss's five steps in Selective coding are absolutely not necessary and that steps 2 and 3 force the data into the coding paradigm, rather than allowing emergence to happen.<br><br>• Argues that the order for developing properties of the core category is opposite that proposed by Strauss. Discovery of properties of a category and its relationship to other categories is how we choose the core category. | • Selective coding is the process of selecting the core category, systematically relating it to other categories, validating those relationships, filling in categories that need further refinement.<br><br>• To systematize and solidify the connections between categories, inductive and deductive thinking is used in a process of reciprocal inductive derivation of categories, and deductively proposing hypotheses to be validated against the data.<br><br>• Choosing the core category can sometimes be difficult and integrating the theory is also hard conceptual work.<br><br>• 5 steps in selective coding: (1) explicating the story line; (2) relating subsidiary categories around the core category via coding paradigm; (3) relating categories at the dimensional level; (4) validating relationships against the data; (5) filling in categories that need refinement (i.e., saturating categories).<br><br>• A core category must be developed in terms of its properties. Once properties are identified, then the next step is relate other categories to it, thus making them subsidiary categories. |

**TABLE 7.1** *(continued)*

| Analytic Category | Glaser (1992) | Strauss & Corbin (1990) |
|---|---|---|
| Process | • Glaser agrees with Strauss' initial statement on process.<br>• He disagrees with the need to attend to process by noting the changes because this is preconceiving and forcing the data yet again into the 6C coding family.<br>• Glaser says that process is only elusive because Strauss has not stuck to the original definition of process as a set of stages that can be conceptually named. Glaser says that process will naturally emerge if and when it is relevant or the prime mover of participants. If a person does not refer to process, it isn't relevant. If the analyst needs to account for change by attending to process that is not emerging in the data, then this is forcing.<br>• Glaser argues that non-progressive movement is not a useful analytic concept; it does not neatly "order out." For Glaser, process is linear. | • Process is the linking of action/interactional sequences as they pertain to the management of, control over or response to a phenomenon and needs to be attended to in GT. Linking sequences is done by noting, (a) change in conditions over time, (b) action/interactional response to the change, (c) the consequences that result, and (d) how consequences become part of conditions influencing next action/interactional sequence.<br>• Strauss argues that process is an elusive term that does not necessarily stand out in the data. Process does not always just emerge (although it should), but unless the analyst identifies it and builds it into the analysis it might be missed. It may be necessary to theoretically sample for it and go back to the field.<br>• Strauss says process is the analyst's way of accounting for change because a participant often does not refer to process in terms of phases or stages.<br>• When change is noticed in the data, one analyzes it in terms of specific properties.<br>• Process can be either progressive or non-progressive movement (i.e., stages/phases versus non-linear sequencing). |

*(continued)*

**TABLE 7.1** *(continued)*

| Analytic Category | Glaser (1992) | Strauss & Corbin (1990) |
|---|---|---|
| Conditional Matrix | • Glaser does not see GT as a "transactional system." He denies categorically that all phenomena are embedded in sets of conditions. He also denies Strauss's statement that conditions at all levels have relevance for any study.<br><br>• Glaser completely rejects the conditional matrix because it preconceives the data. To use the matrix, Glaser says one has to force the data into it because levels of analysis are not always important.<br><br>• The terminology is foreign to grounded theory. He argues that these concepts are used to develop, not to discover conditions and consequences at all levels. | • The conditional matrix is a transactional analysis system used as an analytic aid to considering the wide range of conditions and consequences related to the phenomenon under study. It is conceptualized as nested concentric circles, each representing a level of analysis. A phenomenon itself will be embedded in a specific level of the matrix.<br><br>• At the center of the matrix is action/interaction pertaining to a phenomenon. The layers range from individual, group, community, organizational, through to national and international.<br><br>• It is seen as aiding theoretical sensitivity to identifying the conditions that might impinge on the action/interaction in relation to the phenomenon under study.<br><br>• All phenomena are assumed to be embedded in sets of conditions.<br><br>• The researcher needs to fill in the specific conditional features for each level that pertain to the area. Conditions may emerge from the data, or could come from researcher experience, or the literature. BUT, they are provisional and must earn their way into the data. |

**TABLE 7.1** *(continued)*

| Analytic Category | Glaser (1992) | Strauss & Corbin (1990) |
|---|---|---|
| Theoretical Sampling | • Glaser objects to the notion of fracturing the concept of theoretical sampling into the different types, which he says is unnecessary. Also, because he does not do axial coding, the sampling related to axial coding would be irrelevant to him.<br><br>• Glaser criticizes this aim because he argues that preconceptions will drive sampling decisions rather than the data themselves. | • Theoretical sampling is on the basis of concepts with theoretical relevance to the evolving theory. Three types of theoretical sampling:<br><br>1. Open sampling—associated with open coding, in which openness rather than specificity guides the choices<br>2. Relational and Variational Sampling—associated with Axial coding, aimed at finding differences at the dimensional level<br>3. Discriminant Sampling—associated with selective coding. Aim is to maximize opportunities for verifying the story line<br><br>• The aim in theoretical sampling is to sample incidents, not persons, to gather data about action/interaction, conditions giving rise to action, how conditions change or stay the same, and the consequences (i.e., in terms of the coding paradigm). |

# REFERENCES

Alexander, J., Giesen, B., Münch, R., & Smelser, N. (1987). *The macro-micro link*. Berkeley: University of California Press.

Annells, M. (1996). Grounded theory method: Philosophical perspectives, paradigm of inquiry, and postmodernism. *Qualitative Health Research, 6*, 379–393.

Antonio, R. J. (1989). The normative foundations of emancipatory theory: Evolutionary versus pragmatic perspectives. *American Journal of Sociology, 94*, 721–748.

Ashton, J., & Seymour, H. (1988). *The new public health*. Milton Keynes: Open University Press.

Blumer, H. (1937). Social psychology. In E. Schmidt (Ed.), *Man and society* (pp. 144–198). New York: Prentice-Hall.

Blumer, H. (1969). *Symbolic interactionism: Perspective and method*. Englewood Cliffs, NJ: Prentice-Hall.

Bunton, R., & Macdonald, G. (1992). *Health promotion: Disciplines and diversity*. London: Routledge.

Butterfield, P. G. (1990). Thinking upstream: Nurturing a conceptual understanding of the societal context of health behavior. *Advances in Nursing Science, 12*(2), 1–8.

Clarke, H., & Mass, H. (1998). Comox Valley Nursing Centre: From collaboration to empowerment. *Public Health Nursing, 15*(3), 216–224.

Cook, T. D. (1985). Postpositivist critical multiplism. In R. L. Shotland & M. Mark (Eds.), *Social science and social policy* (pp. 21–62). Beverly Hills, CA: Sage Publications.

Denzin, N. K. (1992). *Symbolic interactionism and cultural studies*. Oxford, UK: Blackwell.

Dewey, J. (1922). *Human nature and conduct*. New York: Holt.

Duncan, S. M. (1996). Empowerment strategies in nursing education: A foundation for population focused clinical studies. *Public Health Nursing, 13*(5), 311–317.

Glaser, B. (1978). *Theoretical sensitivity*. Mill Valley, CA: Sociology Press.

Glaser, B. (1992). *Basics of grounded theory analysis*. Mill Valley, CA: Sociology Press.

Glaser, B. (1998). *Doing grounded theory: Issues and discussions*. Mill Valley, CA: Sociology Press.

Glaser, B., & Strauss, A. (1967). *The discovery of grounded theory*. Chicago: Aldine.

Glaser, B., & Strauss, A. (1968). *A time for dying*. Chicago: Aldine.

Green, L. W., Richard, L., & Potvin, L. (1996). Ecological foundations of health promotion. *American Journal of Health Promotion, 10*, 270–281.

Guba, E. G., & Lincoln, Y. S. (1989). *Fourth generation evaluation.* Newbury Park: Sage Publications.

Guba, E. G., & Lincoln, Y. S. (1994). Competing paradigms in qualitative research. In N. K. Denzin & Y. S. Lincoln (Eds.), *Handbook of qualitative research* (pp. 104–117). Thousand Oaks, CA: Sage Publications.

Habermas, J. (1987). *The theory of communicative action* (2nd ed.). Boston: Beacon Press.

Henwood, K., & Pidgeon, N. (1995). Remaking the link: Qualitative research and feminist standpoint theory. *Feminism & Psychology, 5*(1), 7–30.

Huber, J. (1974). The emergency of emergent theory. *American Sociological Review, 39,* 463–466.

Hutchinson, S. (1986). Grounded theory: The method. In P. Munhall & C. Oiler (Eds.), *Nursing research: A qualitative perspective* (pp. 111–129). Connecticut: Appleton-Century Crofts.

Kendall, J. (1992). Fighting back: Promoting emancipatory nursing actions. *Advances in Nursing Science, 15*(2), 1–15.

Kulbok, P., Baldwin, J. H., Cox, C. L., & Duffy, R. (1997). Advancing discourse on health promotion: Beyond mainstream thinking. *Advances in Nursing Science, 20*(1), 12–20.

Layder, D. (1982). Grounded theory: A constructive critique. *Journal for Theory in Social Behaviour, 12,* 102–123.

Layder, D. (1989a). *New strategies in social research.* Cambridge, UK: Polity Press.

Layder, D. (1989b). The macro-micro distinction, social relations, and methodological bracketing. *Current Perspectives in Social Theory, 9,* 123–141.

Lowenburg, J. S. (1995). Health promotion and the "ideology of choice." *Public Health Nursing, 12*(5), 319–323.

Maben, J., & MacLeod Clark, J. (1995). Health promotion: A concept analysis. *Journal of Advanced Nursing, 22,* 1158–1165.

MacDonald, M. (in press). Health promotion: Historical, theoretical, and philosophical perspectives. In L. E. Young & V. Hayes (Eds.), *Transforming health promotion practice: Concepts, issues and applications.* Philadelphia: F. A. Davis.

Maines, D. (1993). Foreword. In A. Strauss, *Continual permutations of action* (pp. xiii–xv). New York: Aldine de Gruyter.

Maxwell, L. E. (1997). Foundational thought in the development of knowledge for social change. In S. Thorne & V. Hayes (Eds.), *Nursing praxis: Knowledge and action* (pp. 203–218). Thousand Oaks: Sage Publications.

Melia, K. M. (1996). Rediscovering Glaser. *Qualitative Health Research, 6,* 368–378.

Meltzer, B. N., & Herman, N. J. (1990). Epilogue: Human emotion, social structure and symbolic interactionism. In L. Reynolds (Ed.), *Interactionism: Exposition and critique* (2nd ed.) (pp. 181–225). Dix Hills, NY: Great Hall, Inc.

Münch, R. (1994). *Sociological theory: From the 1850s to the 1920s.* Chicago: Nelson Hall Publishers.

Novak, J. (1988). The social mandate and historical basis for nursing's role in health promotion. *Journal of Professional Nursing, 4*(2), 80–87.

Park, R. E., Burgess, E. W., & McKenzie, R. D. (Eds.). (1925). *The city.* Chicago: University of Chicago Press.

Pender, N. (1987). *Health promotion in nursing practice* (2nd ed.). Stamford, CT: Appleton & Lange.

Pender, N. (1996). *Health promotion in nursing practice* (3rd ed.). Stamford, CT: Appleton & Lange.

Poland, B. D. (1992). Learning to "walk our talk": The implications of sociological theory for research methodologies in health promotion. *Canadian Journal of Public Health, 83,* S31–S46.

Prendergast, C., & Knotternerus, J. D. (1993). The new studies in social organization: Overcoming the structural bias. In L. T. Reynolds (Ed.), *Interactionism: Expostion and critique* (3rd ed.). Dix Hills, NY: General Hall, Inc.

Reynolds, L. T. (1993). *Interactionism: Exposition and critique* (3rd ed.). Dix Hills, NY: General Hall, Inc.

Robertson, A., & Minkler, M. (1994). A new health promotion movement: A critical examination. *Health Education Quarterly, 21,* 295–312.

Rush, K. (1997). Health promotion ideology and nursing education. *Journal of Advanced Nursing, 25,* 1292–1298.

Schatzman, L. (1991). Dimensional analysis: Notes on an alternative approach to the grounding of theory in qualitative research. In D. R. Maines (Ed.), *Social organization and social process: Essays in honor of Anselm Strauss* (pp. 303–314). New York: Aldine de Gruyter.

Shalin, D. N. (1992). Critical theory and the pragmatist challenge. *American Journal of Sociology, 98,* 237–279.

Stanley, L., & Wise, S. (1983). *Breaking out: Feminist consciousness and feminist research.* London: Routledge and Kegan Paul.

Stern, P. N. (1994). Eroding grounded theory. In J. M. Morse (Ed.), *Critical issues in qualitative research methods* (pp. 212–223). Thousand Oaks: Sage Publications.

Stevens, P. E. (1989). A critical social reconceptualization of environment in nursing: Implications for methodology. *Advances in Nursing Science, 11*(4), 56–68.

Stevens, P. E., & Hall, J. (1992). Applying critical theories to nursing in communities. *Public Health Nursing, 9*(1), 2–9.

Stokols, D. (1992). Establishing and maintaining healthy environments: Toward a social ecology of health promotion. *American Psychologist, 47*, 6–22.

Strauss, A. (1959/1969). *Mirrors and masks.* San Francisco: Sociology Press.

Strauss, A. (1978). *Negotiations.* San Francisco: Jossey Bass.

Strauss, A. (1987). *Qualitative methods for social scientists.* Cambridge: Cambridge University Press.

Strauss, A. L. (1993). *Continual permutations of action.* New York: Aldine de Gruyter.

Strauss, A., & Corbin, J. (1990). *Basics of qualitative research: Grounded theory procedures and techniques.* Newbury Park, CA: Sage Publications.

Strauss, A., & Corbin, J. (1994). Grounded theory methodology: An overview. In N. K. Denzin & Y. S. Lincoln (Eds.), *Handbook of qualitative research* (pp. 273–285). Thousand Oaks, CA: Sage Publications.

Strauss, A. J., & Corbin, J. (1998). *Basics of qualitative research: Techniques and procedures for developing grounded theory.* Thousand Oaks, CA: Sage.

Vaughn, T. R., & Reynolds, L. T. (1968). The sociology of symbolic interactionism. *American Sociologist, 3*, 208–214.

Williams, D. M. (1989). Political theory and individualistic health promotion. *Advances in Nursing Science, 12(1)*, 14–25.

World Health Organization. (1986). *Ottawa Charter for health promotion.* Ottawa: Canadian Public Health Association & Health and Welfare Canada.

Wuest, J. (1995). Feminist grounded theory: An exploration of the congruency and tensions between two traditions in knowledge discovery. *Qualitative Health Research, 5*(1), 125–137.

shaped *but not completely defined* by the process through which it was created. (1994, p. 14)

Many would-be grounded theorists produce "theories" that are mere descriptions and stop short of constructing a full representation of participants' reality (Stern, 1994; Wilson & Hutchinson, 1996). A fully developed grounded theory goes beyond the mundane data and description to an evocative and elegant explanation of that reality in a way that is immediately recognizable to those in the know (May, 1994; Sandelowski, 1994). A grounded theory without these qualities cannot meet the basic requirements for scientific rigor in grounded theory, that is, fit, work, and grab (Glaser, 1978). Until the theorist has constructed a symbolic representation that explains the relationships among concepts and illuminates the actions and interactions of participants, the data are not sufficiently analyzed nor the theory fully developed. What results is a description, not a theory, and certainly not a grounded theory. Without magic in the analytical method, grounded theory is reduced to a mere set of techniques, and the result lacks the characteristic gestalt that defines a grounded theory.

## CONCLUSION

To return to our question, can you "do" grounded theory without symbolic interactionism? Certainly, some of the individual techniques, such as constant comparison, can be used freely, however, we suggest that grounded theory is more than the sum of its techniques. Even if we consider grounded theory as merely a set of techniques, it is evident to us that these techniques embrace key elements of symbolic interactionism.

As illustrated in Figure 9.1, symbolic interactionism penetrates even the technical level of grounded theory so that, in our view, an adequate grounded theory study cannot be divorced from it. Even the grounded theory researcher who is unfamiliar with symbolic interactionism *per se* is necessarily enacting the epistemological underpinnings of the method through the conduct of her or his study.

Nonetheless, just as a grounded theory is more than a description of the data, grounded theory as a method is more than the tasks

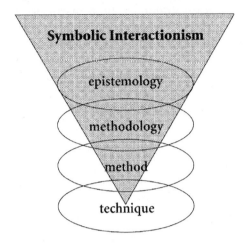

**FIGURE 9.1** **The relationship between symbolic interactionism and grounded theory.**

performed by the researcher. Grounded theory research must result in a parsimonious, evocative construction that illuminates and explains the actions and interactions of participants as they manage the basic social problem. To achieve this end, the researcher necessarily engages in symbolic interaction—within herself or himself, with the data, with participants, and with the emerging theory. Thus, for us, grounded theory is a comprehensive package, not simply a set of techniques. Anything short of this, purporting to be a grounded theory, fails to achieve accepted standards of rigor in grounded theory and is simply bad science. As Sandelowski (1994) says, the proof is in the pottery.

Thus, it is our view that symbolic interactionism is inherent in grounded theory research, whether the researcher is aware of it or not. If research is truly grounded theory, it cannot occur in the absence of symbolic interactionism, which is intrinsic to the process. This does not imply that other theoretical perspectives, such as feminism (see Wuest & Merritt-Gray, chapter 8, this volume), critical theory (see MacDonald, chapter 7, this volume), or hermeneutics (see Pursley-Crotteau, Bunting, & Draucker, chapter 10, this volume) may not be incorporated as well, but that these other perspectives are superimposed onto symbolic interactionism. In these circumstances, the researcher is challenged to reconcile the ontological and epistemological stances of these differing perspectives.

Thus, for us, grounded theory is both a method and a methodology, and contains within it its own philosophical justification. This should not be surprising, as any research method is imbued with an epistemology that guides its unfolding. For example, statistical research is based on positivist and post-positivist assumptions about the nature of knowledge, what can be known, who can know it, and how it can be studied. Consequently, there is an unarticulated epistemology underpinning SPSS. As Denzin (1972) noted, " . . . methods are not atheoretical tools, but rather means of acting on the environment and making that environment meaningful" (p. 77). We share Denzin's view.

## REFERENCES

Abercrombie, N., Hill, S., & Turner, B. S. (1984). *The Penguin dictionary of sociology*. Middlesex, UK: Penguin Books.

Barnhart, C. L. (1970). *The American college dictionary*. New York: Random House.

Blumer, H. (1954). What is wrong with social theory? *American Sociological Review, 19*, 3–18.

Blumer, H. (1969/1986). *Symbolic interactionism: Perspective and method*. Berkeley, CA: University of California Press.

Campbell, J. C., & Bunting, S. (1991). Voices and paradigms: Perspectives on critical and feminist theory in nursing. *Advances in Nursing Science, 13*(3), 1–15.

Denzin, N. (1972). The research act: The interrelationship of theory & method. In J. G. Manis & B. N. Meltzer (Eds.), *Symbolic interaction: A reader in social psychology*, 2nd ed. (pp. 76–91). Boston: Allyn & Bacon, Inc.

Dey, I. (1999). *Grounding grounded theory: Guidelines for qualitative inquiry*. Toronto, ON: Academic Press.

Glaser, B. G. (1978). *Theoretical sensitivity*. Mill Valley, CA: Sociology Press.

Glaser, B. (1998). Doing grounded theory: Issues and discussions. Mill Valley, CA: Sociology Press.

Glaser, B. G. (1999). The future of grounded theory. *Qualitative Health Research, 9*(6), 836–845.

Glaser, B. G., & Strauss, A. (1967). *The discovery of grounded theory.* Chicago: Aldine.

Guba, E. G., & Lincoln, Y. S. (1989). *Fourth generation evaluation.* Newbury Park, CA: Sage.

Harding, S. (1987). Introduction: Is there a feminist model? In S. Harding (Ed.), *Feminism and methodology* (pp. 1–14). Bloomington, IN: Indiana University Press.

Kaplan, A. (1964). *The conduct of inquiry: Methodology for behavioral science.* San Francisco: Chandler Publishing.

Kirby, S., & McKenna, K. (1989). *Experience, research, social change: Methods from the margins.* Toronto: Garamond.

Konecki, K. (1989). The methodology of grounded theory in the research of the situation of work. *The Polish Sociological Bulletin, 2,* 59–74.

Manis, J. G., & Meltzer, B. N. (1972). Intellectual antecedents and basic propositions of symbolic interactionsim. In J. Manis & B. Meltzer (Eds.), *Symbolic interaction: A reader in social psychology* (pp. 1–10). Boston: Allyn and Bacon.

May, K. A. (1994). Abstract knowing: The case for magic in method. In J. M. Morse (Ed.), *Critical issues in qualitative research methods* (pp. 10–21). Thousand Oaks, CA: Sage.

Morgan, D. L. (1998). *The focus group guidebook.* Thousand Oaks, CA: Sage.

Munhall, P. L. (1993). Epistemology in nursing. In P. L. Munhall & C. O. Boyd (Eds.), *Nursing research: A qualitative perspective* (pp. 39–65). New York: National League for Nursing Press.

Sandelowski, M. (1994). The proof is in the pottery: Toward a poetic for qualitative inquiry. In J. M. Morse (Ed.), *Critical issues in qualitative research methods* (pp. 46–63). Thousand Oaks, CA: Sage.

Schwandt, T. A. (1994). Constructivist, interpretivist approaches to human inquiry. In N. K. Denzin & Y. S. Lincoln (Eds.), *Handbook of qualitative research* (pp. 118–137). Thousand Oaks, CA: Sage.

Stern, P. N. (1994). Eroding grounded theory. In J. M. Morse (Ed.), *Critical issues in qualitative research methods* (pp. 212–223). Thousand Oaks, CA: Sage.

Wilson, H. S., & Hutchinson, S. A. (1996). Methodologic mistakes in grounded theory. *Nursing Research, 45*(2), 122–124.

# CHAPTER 10

# Grounded Theory and Hermeneutics: Contradictory or Complementary Methods of Nursing Research?

**Suzanne Pursley-Crotteau,
Sheila McGuire Bunting, and
Claire Burke Draucker**

Grounded theory and hermeneutics are interpretive methods frequently used in qualitative nursing research. Grounded theory is a research approach used to generate substantive theory of basic social or social-psychological processes experienced by groups who share a common problem or concern. Hermeneutics is a research approach used to discover meaning and achieve understanding of everyday lived experiences. Both methods are considered phenomenological as they are used to describe the worlds of persons being studied (Stern, 1994). Researchers using these methods share several common beliefs and practices: they view knowledge as tentative and evolving, produce findings that are a result of an interpretive collaboration between researcher and participant, and seek to answer research questions that inform practice (Baker, Norton, Young, & Ward, 1998). The ontological and epistemological assumptions on which the two methods are based, however, are distinct. Grounded theory is rooted in symbolic interactionism (Blumer, 1969; Mead, 1934/1962) and hermeneutics is rooted in the philosophy of phenomenology (Dilthey, 1990; Gadamer, 1975; Heidegger, 1962).

Wilson and Hutchinson (1991) advocated the triangulation of grounded theory and Heideggerian hermeneutics to understand complex human phenomena and to provide "the breadth and depth needed in nursing science" (p. 275). They argued that hermeneutics can provide rich detail that can inform how we think about our practice, whereas grounded theory can yield a conceptual framework on which to base interventions. Some researchers have suggested, however, that the different philosophical groundings of the two methods make it difficult to espouse both paradigms (Darbyshire, 1994). Indeed, since the Wilson and Hutchinson article was published, few researchers have accepted the challenge to triangulate both methods and for good reason. Triangulation was originally a technical term used in surveying and navigation to describe the technique of using two known or visible points to plot the location of a third point (Knafl & Breitmayer, 1991). Social scientists initially used it metaphorically to characterize the use of multiple methods to measure the same construct (Campbell, 1956; Campbell & Fiske, 1959). Researchers later expanded the use of triangulation to include the use of quantitative and qualitative methods. The appropriateness of the use of both methods in the same research project stimulated much debate and discussion (Flick, 1992; Goodwin & Goodwin, 1994), but this has not daunted its use in nursing and behavioral sciences. Researchers have also suggested that the different philosophical perspectives of grounded theory and hermeneutics make it difficult to espouse both paradigms (Darbyshire, 1994). In this chapter, we review and compare the historical roots, the methodological perspectives, and the analytic procedures of the two approaches in order to consider whether they can be successfully triangulated, as suggested by Wilson and Hutchinson, or whether to do so would threaten the integrity of both methods. A study that used both grounded theory and hermeneutics to study women's responses to violence will be described.

# GROUNDED THEORY

## Historical Roots

Grounded theory is rooted in symbolic interactionism, which focuses on the meaning of events to people in natural settings. Social interactionism is derived from the work of pragmatic philosophers such as John Dewey and William James. The basic propositions of pragmatic philosophy are:

1. Truth does not exist "out there" in the real world but is actively created as humans act toward the world;
2. People base their knowledge of the world on what has proven useful to them;
3. People define the social and physical objects they encounter in the world according to the way they can use them; and
4. If we want to understand people, we must understand what those people do in the world and how they interpret that world (Ritzer, 1983).

Symbolic interactionism was developed by George Herbert Mead who taught philosophy at the University of Chicago from 1894 to 1931. Mead's major work was *Mind, Self, and Society: From the Standpoint of a Social Behaviorist* (Mead, 1934/1962). Herbert Blumer (1969) refined Mead's propositions. According to Blumer, symbolic interactionism is based on three basic principles:

1. Human beings act toward things on the basis of the meanings that things have for them;
2. Meaning of such things is derived from, or arises out of, the social interaction that one has with one's fellows; and
3. These meanings are handled in, and modified through, an interpretative process used by the person in dealing with the things she or he encounters (Blumer, 1969, p. 2).

All human behavior is considered "a vast interpretive process in which people, singly and collectively, guide themselves by defining the objects, events and situations they encounter" (Blumer, 1969, p. 132). From the symbolic interaction perspective, behavior is studied on two levels: the behavioral or interactional, and the symbolic. Through social interaction, individuals are always designating symbols to each other and to themselves (Bowers, 1988). With its roots in pragmatism and social interactionism, grounded theory has as its purpose the derivation of theory that explains the interactions of people within a given context. The researcher asks and answers the question, "What are the processes and meanings people use to manage their worlds?"

## Methodological Perspective

Grounded theory was explicated by Glaser and Strauss in *The Discovery of Grounded Theory* (1967). The primary purposes of this work were to offer a rationale for theory developed through interplay with data collected in research, suggest the logic for and specifics of grounded theories, and legitimize qualitative research through adequate verification (Strauss & Corbin, 1994, p. 275). Glaser (1978) suggested that grounded theory could be used by any discipline interested in "generating theory and doing social research as two parts of the same process" (Glaser, 1978, p. 2).

In grounded theory, the researcher seeks to understand the actions of the individual or collective actors under study and to account for change over time. Sources of data may include interviews and field observations, videotapes, letters, diaries, autobiographies, biographies, newspapers, and other media materials. The researcher can also use quantitative data or a combination of qualitative and quantitative data for the analysis. The perspectives and voices of the participants are included in the study findings. Although the grounded theory researcher carefully examines and considers the participants' expressed meanings, he or she assumes final responsibility for the interpretation. The findings reflect the theoretical formulation developed by the researcher. Grounded theory procedures are considered amenable to different levels of theory development from substantive theory to general formal theories (Glaser, 1978; Strauss & Corbin, 1994).

## Analytic Procedures

Although grounded theory was designed to allow for much latitude and ingenuity by the researcher (Strauss & Corbin, 1994), analytic procedures have been prescribed. The constant comparison of concepts derived from the data is the main analytic process used in grounded theory (Glaser & Strauss, 1967). Analysis begins with open coding of the data in which interview texts and other documents are coded word-by-word and line-by-line to completely open or "fracture" the data. Substantive coding then includes the processes of developing categories and relating the categories to one another in theoretical statements. The researcher then returns to the data to establish validity of these statements by finding confirming or contrary instances.

The researcher may seek additional data in the forms of a literature review, interviews of new participants, or additional interviews of previous participants. This process of seeking data from various sources to confirm or offer contrary cases of the theoretical statements is called theoretical sampling, the hallmark of the grounded theory method. Using theoretical sampling, the researcher allows the emerging theory to guide the ongoing sampling process (Glaser, 1978).

Even though these procedures are often described in a linear fashion, the processes of data collection and data analysis are interwoven as the grounded theory is conceptualized. According to Strauss and Corbin (1994), grounded theorists are "much concerned with discovering 'process'—not necessarily in the sense of stages or phases, but of the reciprocal changes in patterns of action/interaction and in relationship with changes of conditions either internal or external to the process itself" (p. 278).

## HERMENEUTICS

### Historical Roots

The term hermeneutics is derived from the Greek word, *hermeneuein,* meaning "to interpret." Originally, hermeneutics was used as a systematic, historical, and critical scientific method specifically for interpreting theological and philosophical exegesis (Welch, 1999).

Friedrich Schleiermacher, a German theologian and philosopher, is considered a creator of modern hermeneutics (Tice, 1995). He first introduced the notion of the hermeneutic circle to reflect the circularity of interpretation; that is, the interpretation of each part of text is dependent on the interpretation of the whole. Because every interpretation is based on another interpretation, one cannot escape the hermeneutic circle (Bohman, 1995).

Dilthey (1900), a German philosopher and historian, was also a significant figure in the development of hermeneutics (Makkreel, 1995). He believed that all human sciences are interpretive and Understanding (with a capital letter) involves the interpretation of expression of human activities, the "objectifications" of life (e.g., literature, art, social life, history) (Polkinghorne, 1983). Understanding is a kind of comprehension that exceeds purely logical analysis through the use of both inductive and deductive logic. Dilthey argued that explanation is the method of the natural sciences and Understanding is the method of the human sciences. Human sciences share the data collection techniques of observation and description with the natural sciences, but add the Understanding or *Verstehen* of human expression through thoughts and emotions. Dilthey believed that both the natural and the humans sciences could obtain objective truth through proper method.

Unlike Dilthey's epistemological perspective, the philosophical hermeneutics of Heidegger (1962) represented an ontological perspective. Heidegger (1962) was a German philosopher who, in his seminal work *Being and Time*, significantly challenged the assumptions of Western science and proposed that being human is being interpretive. Heidegger was interested in the background conditions that enable entities to show up as mattering. To understand why entities are intelligible, one must analyze an entity that has prior understanding, that is, human existence, or *Dasein*. As Guignon (1995) explained:

> Heidegger's claim is that *Dasein's* pretheoretical understanding of being, embodied in its everyday practices, opens a "clearing" in which entities can show up as, say, tools, protons, numbers, mental events, and so on. This historically unfolding clearing is what the metaphysical tradition has overlooked. (p. 317)

For Heidegger, the analytic of *Dasein* involves a description of *Dasein's* everydayness, which is "our ordinary prereflective agency when we are caught up in the midst of our practical affairs" (Guignon, 1995, p. 317) and an account of how understanding is possible. According to Guignon (1995), Heidegger suggested that *Dasein* has three essential structures:

1. Being already in the world. *Dasein* is always already thrown into a world, a concrete historical and social context, to live out its life.
2. Being ahead of itself. *Dasein* is always taking a stance on its life by acting in the world (projection) and is future oriented as its identity is constituted by the ongoing fulfillment of possibilities.
3. Being engaged with things. *Dasein* is always articulating entities that show up in our concernful absorption in current situations (discourse).

Hermeneutics, according to Heidegger, was not a method designed to develop science but rather the very nature of human existence. The hermeneutic question is: "What does it mean to be?" Understanding is not a way of knowing, but a mode of being—our basic way of our "being in the world."

Gadamer (1975), a German philosopher who was strongly influenced by Heidegger, believed that hermeneutics is the most fundamental aspect of all disciplines (Koch, 1996) and discussed several important concepts related to interpretation. In his book *Truth and Method*, Gadamer discussed the concept of prejudice, which he defined as "a judgment that is given before all elements that determine a situation have been fully examined" (p. 270). All interpreters have expectations based on their own beliefs, practices, and values. Gadamer also introduced the notion of the fusion of horizons, a metaphor for understanding. Koch (1996) explained:

> Fusion is the coming together of different vantage points. The process leading to fusion of horizons is . . . like a posture, or a way of conducting yourself, a willingness to open yourself to the standpoint of another so that you can let their standpoint speak to you, and let it influence you. (p. 177)

For both Heidegger and Gadamer, therefore, true understanding is the consequence of human engagement; there is no "pure truth."

## Methodological Perspectives

While hermeneutics as a contemporary research method is based primarily on the ontological philosophies of Heidegger and Gadamer, Heidegger considered his project to be one of philosophical reflection; he rebelled against the notion of "method" and the term "research" (Cohen & Omery, 1994). Gadamer (1975) also was not interested in describing a methodological procedure for the human sciences (Annells, 1996). As Cohen and Omery (1994) stressed, "It fell on others to define what the hermeneutic was to become as a research method" (p. 147).

Van Manen (1990) outlined six research activities that are critical to the interpretive endeavor:

1. Turning to a phenomenon, which seriously interests us and commits us to the world;
2. Investigating experience as we live it rather than as we conceptualize it;
3. Reflecting on essential themes, which characterize the phenomenon;
4. Describing the phenomenon through the art of writing and rewriting;
5. Maintaining a strong and oriented pedagogical relation to the phenomenon;
6. Balancing the research context by considering parts and whole. (pp. 30–31)

Research based on hermeneutic, or interpretive, phenomenology, is often contrasted with research based on eidectic, or descriptive, phenomenology (Cohen & Omery, 1994). As a research method, eidectic phenomenology is based on the assumption that all human experience has essential structures that take on meaning when consciously apprehended. The goal of this method is a description of the meaning of experience from the perspective or worldview of those who have the experience. "Researchers bracket their presuppositions, reflect on the experiences that were described, and intuit or describe the essential structures of the experiences under study" (Cohen & Omery, 1994, p. 148).

In contrast, hermeneutics as a research method rests on the ontological assumption that all experience is an interpretive process. The purpose of hermeneutic research is interpretation and understanding of a lived experience—to understand what it means to be a person in the world (Walters, 1995). Researchers do not attempt to suspend the presuppositions they bring to the research, rather they examine them as part of the interpretive process. In hermeneutical inquiry, "the data generated by the participants is fused with the experience of the researchers and placed in context" (Koch, 1996, p. 176).

Hermeneutic researchers may utilize many sources of data, including individual and group interviews, participant observation, videotapes, documents, public writings, and media (Benner, 1994). When talking with participants, interviewers ask for narrative accounts of specific experiences, rather than ideas or opinions about certain issues. Second interviews are recommended to give the researcher and participant a chance to ensure that understanding has occurred.

## Analytic Procedures

Although those who write about hermeneutic research stress that there are no cookbook recipes to guide analysis, some practical guidelines, typically aimed at novice researchers, have been explicated. Benner (1985), for example, described the basic process of hermeneutic analysis:

> Interview material and observations are turned into text through transcription. The interpretation entails a systematic analysis of the whole text, a systematic analysis of parts of the text, and a comparison of the two interpretations for conflicts and for understanding the whole in relation to the parts, and vice versa. Whole cases may be compared to whole cases. Usually, this shifting back and forth between the parts and the whole reveals new themes, new issues, and new questions that are generated in the process of understanding the text itself. (p. 9)

Three interpretive and presentation strategies are recommended for interpretive study (Benner, 1985). Paradigm cases are whole cases that are clear and vivid examples of a particular pattern of meaning. Exemplars are parts of text, such as stories or vignettes, that demonstrate concerns and practices within context. A thematic analysis is the identification of themes in the data that represent common meanings.

The most frequently employed application of the hermeneutic philosophical premises to a research method was explicated by Diekelmann, Allen, and Tanner (1989). These authors have delineated the steps of the process of analysis for hermeneutics. Researchers, who often work in teams, read each interview to obtain an overall understanding, write interpretive summaries of each interview, and code for possible themes. Transcripts are then analyzed by the group to develop the themes. Analysts continually return to the text or to the participants for clarification and understanding, always moving back and forth from the whole of the text to the specific textual examples to aid in interpretation. A composite analysis of each text is written. Texts are then compared and contrasted to identify and describe shared practices and common meanings across texts. The team identifies constitutive patterns and connections across themes and collaborates on a final draft of the findings.

Benner (1995) argued that when one gains skills in interpretive work, the need for rules falls away. She stated, "Indeed, as Dreyfus (1991) contends, models (and rules) would not even work to capture the know-how of skilled involvement in the world that Heidegger calls the ready-to-hand mode of engagement, that is, the smooth functioning of expertise or understanding" (p. 78).

## RESEARCH TRIANGULATING HEIDEGGERIAN HERMENEUTICS AND GROUNDED THEORY: WOMEN'S RESPONSES TO SEXUAL VIOLENCE BY MALE INTIMATES

Draucker (Draucker & Madsen, 1999; Draucker & Stern, 2000) conducted a study using both Heideggerian hermeneutics and grounded theory to explore women's responses to sexual violence by male intimates. The study was an Academic Investigator Award program funded by the National Institute of Nursing Research. The author's mentors for the project were Drs. Phyllis Stern and Nancy Diekelmann. The aims of the study were to:

1. obtain descriptions of (a) the meaning of violence in their current lives, and (b) their day-to-day experiences of being a

survivor of violence from women who have experienced sexual violence within an intimate relationship in adulthood;

2. analyze and present these descriptions using hermeneutic methods;
3. obtain descriptions of healing experiences from women who have experienced healing from sexual violence within an intimate relationship in adulthood;
4. construct a theoretical framework outlining the process of healing from intimate sexual violence using the grounded theory method;
5. combine the findings on surviving and healing to provide a comprehensive description of women's responses to the experience of living through intimate sexual violence;
6. develop recommendations for nursing interventions for women who have survived intimate sexual violence in adulthood, based on the results of this project and current knowledge in the field.

Aims 1 and 2 were achieved by a Heideggerian hermeneutic study of 10 women who had experienced sexual violence by a male intimate, and aims 3 and 4 were achieved by a grounded theory study of 33 women who had experienced some healing from an experience of sexual violence by a male intimate. Aims 5 and 6 were achieved by merging the findings of both approaches. As recommended by Wilson and Hutchinson (1991), the samples were kept separate "to remain true to the tenets of both methods" (p. 269) and the focus of the interviews was different. The women in Study A were asked to describe their day-to-day experiences of being a survivor of violence, and women in Study B were asked to describe how their lives had progressed since the time of the violence. The interviews lasted between 1 and 3 hours. Many women maintained contact with the investigator throughout the course of the project, providing additional data via phone contacts or written correspondence.

## Study A: Heideggerian Hermeneutics

The data provided by the 10 women in Study A were analyzed using hermeneutical methods, similar to those outlined by Diekelmann,

Allen, and Tanner (1989). Two themes that emerged from the data were explored using the participants' text, Heideggerian philosophy, and other literature sources.

### Dwelling with Violence

The first theme, dwelling with violence, reflects the women's descriptions of living among and inseparable from violence, abuse, and maltreatment (Draucker & Madsen, 1999). Early in the interpretive process, it was clear that the women's stories were not about a single episode of sexual violence or an abusive relationship, but rather about multiple and varied experiences of violence throughout their lives (e.g., childhood abuse, physical violence in adult relationships, sexual exploitation at school and/or work, fear from living in everyday environments that are dangerous or hostile to women). The Heideggerian concept of dwelling helped deepen our understanding of the participants' experiences as ways of "being in" a violent world. Heidegger (1971), in his essay "Building Dwelling Thinking," argued that to be human means to dwell (*bauen*) on earth as a mortal. The nature of dwelling is remaining or staying in place. Dwelling is experienced as *wunian*, which means "to be at peace, to be brought to peace, to stay at peace" (p. 149). The word for peace (*friede*) is to be preserved from harm and danger, to spare. Dwelling with violence is the "remaining or staying in place, finding peace, and being preserved from harm and danger" when these essential ways of being-in-the-world are challenged by violence, abuse, and maltreatment.

Two experiences related to dwelling were revealed in the texts. Violence resulted in the women "living-in-exile"—feeling uprooted, unsettled, unprotected, and distrustful. Yet, their stories were about "preserving and sparing amidst violence"—caring for the things they valued, creating a safe place for themselves, guarding those things which are essential to their nature, and seeking to protect others.

### Knowing What to Do

The second theme, knowing what to do, reflects the women's descriptions of how they intuitively knew how to manage their lives during and after their violent experiences by using practical, commonsense activities (Draucker, 1999a). The women gave examples of knowing how to do things to survive the violence (e.g., intuitively knowing whether to fight or resist), to attempt to stay safe (e.g., "scoping out" potentially dangerous men), and to make things better (e.g., reading, keeping journals).

The Heideggerian concept of understanding as know-how was used to interpret the women's narratives. Their narratives reflected Heidegger's concept of understanding as a basic way of being in the world (knowing how) rather than a cognitive process (knowing what). In *Being and Time*, Heidegger (1927/1962) stated that "when we are talking ontically we sometimes use the expression 'understanding something' with the signification of 'being able to manage something,' 'being a match for it,' 'being competent to do something' " (p. 183). For women who had experienced violence, being-in-the-world entails "being a match for" the suffering created by violence.

The issue of thrownness (as described above) was also evident in the women's narratives. Many discussed familial and social worlds (e.g., abusive parents, an oppressive society) that both created and limited their possibilities. *Speilrum* (translated as room for maneuver) is that which "permits particular coping activities to show up as possible in the current world" (Dreyfus, 1995, p. 186). Room for maneuver is the range of possibilities in a given circumstance, one's leeway. This nonreflective understanding of what makes sense in a certain circumstance was reflected in the women's beliefs that they knew what to do and the practical, commonsense activities they used to manage the violence and its aftermath.

## Study B: Grounded Theory

Data provided by the 33 women in this phase were used to construct a theoretical framework using grounded theory methods (Draucker & Stern, 2000). Originally, we asked each woman to reflect on her healing from the violence, but several rejected the term healing, stating instead that they had simply struggled to get on with their daily lives. In subsequent interviews, therefore, we asked the women to describe the violence and how their lives had progressed since the violence.

We identified and labeled the core variable as "forging ahead in a dangerous world." This variable represented the women's struggles to get on with their daily lives in a world they knew through firsthand experience to be dangerous.

The women described a wide range of responses to the sexual violence. Their responses were related to their involvement with or commitment to the perpetrator(s) and the extent of violence they had experienced throughout their lives. Therefore, we divided the participants into three groups. Women in Group 1 had experienced a one-time assault; women in Group 2 had experienced sexual violence within abusive relationships; women in Group 3 had experienced a lifetime of abuse and violence. Each group described different variations of forging ahead. Group 1 described *getting back on track;* Group 2 described *starting over again;* and Group 3 described *surviving the long, hard road.* The women in each of the groups discussed three common processes used to forge ahead: *telling others about the violence, making sense of the violence,* and *creating a safer life.*

The nature and function of these processes varied according to group. While all women described telling others about the violence as a way of forging ahead, women in Group 1 needed reassuring talk (revealing the abuse and getting an empathic response); women in Group 2 needed motivating talk (revealing the abuse and being gently challenged to take action, but not pushed to leave the relationship); and women in Group 3 needed restoring talk (revealing the abuse and being given the opportunity to "dig deep" and explore the origins of the violence in their lives).

Similarly, women in the groups differed in how they made sense of the violence. Group 1 women decided they were in the wrong place at the wrong time; Group 2 women figured out why they had chosen "losers"; and Group 3 women came to understand how their bad childhoods had set them up for subsequent violence.

The women created a safer life in different ways as well. Group 1 women used the "wisdom" they acquired from their sexual assault experience to prevent further violence; Group 2 women discovered hidden strengths so they no longer needed "losers" in their lives; and Group 3 women reclaimed their spirit and will to survive. The model suggests that different therapeutic interventions are appropriate for the three groups of women.

Based on the themes identified in Study A and the theoretical framework derived in Study B, recommendations for nursing practice were outlines. The results of these studies, when managed, suggest that health care professionals who work with women who have been sexually assaulted should:

1. Consider the overall effect of violence on women's lives, not just their symptomatic responses to a particular event.
2. Ask about the context of the assault, including the women's relationship and commitment to the perpetrator, societal and family responses to her experience, and her past history of violence.
3. Recognize that women who have endured sexual violence by male intimates face a fundamental paradox. The violent experiences that prompt a search for a safer life are the same experiences that taught them that their social world is dangerous. A treatment approach that focuses not only on the reduction of symptoms but that supports women's attempt to create a safer life is recommended.
4. Consider that women's tacit know-how, if respected and given voice, will ultimately guide their coping. The professional should avoid dictating the survivor's choices or taking action without her consent.
5. Be aware that telling others about experiences of sexual assault or abuse is crucial to recovery—but for different women, different kinds of talk are likely to be helpful. Women who experience single incidents of sexual violence may seek only reassurance and validation, but not advice, from a helping professional; women who experience repeated sexual violence by a partner may profit from talk that "plants the seeds" of change by enhancing their self-esteem without pushing them to leave the relationship; and women who have experienced lifespan abuse need to "dig deep" to explore their past in order to ensure their future.
6. Recognize that finding meaning in an experience of sexual violence is crucial to recovery. Helping professionals, however, should appreciate a woman's need to explain the violence in her own way before they confront any account she holds credible.

7. Consider using a therapeutic approach that elicits women's narratives about how they preserved that which is important to them in order to reveal hidden strengths and competencies.

## CONCLUSION

Hermeneutics and grounded theory methods share several elements. As Wilson and Hutchinson (1991) pointed out, researchers using these methods "share a commitment to a qualitative, naturalistic, contextual, historic, intersubjective methodology to understand human responses and experiences from a variety of perspectives" (p. 267). Yet, there are crucial differences. Interpretive researchers are driven by ontological concerns and enter the hermeneutic circle to achieve understanding and grounded theory researchers are driven by epistemological concerns and analyze field data to develop substantive theory. Differences in research procedures stem from this difference in purpose.

Nurses have consistently employed one method or the other to explore a wide variety of phenomena [see Draucker (1999b) for a review of nursing studies using Heideggerian hermeneutics and Benoliel (1996) for a review of nursing studies using grounded theory], but few have triangulated the two methods. Because we believe that incorporating both perspectives in one project can provide a more holistic view of phenomena of concern (Morse, 1994), we urge researchers to revisit Wilson and Hutchinson's (1991) call to triangulate grounded theory and hermeneutics. In the Draucker project, the hermeneutic study shed light on ways of being in a violent world and the grounded theory study yielded hypotheses with specific implications for practice (i.e., different "types" of violence result in different responses necessitating different therapeutic interventions).

Clearly, there are dangers to triangulation. While both Morse (1994) and Stern (1994) address the potential advantage of using two qualitative methods in the same study, they caution that researchers must keep the analyses separate, avoid "muddling" the methods, and clearly describe the procedures they use. Researchers may assume that, with some adjustment in perspective and "out-of-the-box" thinking, either method can be adapted or mutated. This risks violating the philosophical perspectives and procedures of each method, rendering an "eroded" research product (Baker, Wuest, & Stern, 1992; Stern, 1994).

Triangulation of grounded theory and hermeneutics requires an understanding of and a commitment to the integrity of each tradition, a mentor for each method, collaboration and dialogue with colleagues versed in both approaches, and time (lots of time!). We do believe, however, that such investments may yield fruitful results for nurse researchers.

## REFERENCES

Annells, M. (1996). Hermeneutic phenomenology: Philosophical perspectives and current use in nursing research. *Journal of Advanced Nursing, 23*, 705–713.

Baker, C., Norton, S., Young, P., & Ward, S. (1998). An exploration of methodological pluralism in nursing research. *Research in Nursing and Health, 21*, 545–555.

Baker, C., Wuest, J., & Stern, P. N. (1992). Method slurring: The phenomenology, grounded theory example. *Journal of Advanced Nursing, 1*, 1355–1360.

Benner, P. (1985). Quality of life: A phenomenological perspective on explanation, prediction and understanding in nursing science. *ANS, 8(1)*, 1–14.

Benner, P. (1994). *Interpretive phenomenology: Embodiment, caring, and ethics in health and illness.* Thousand Oaks, CA: Sage.

Benoliel, J. Q. (1996). Grounded theory and nursing knowledge. *Qualitative Health Research, 6(3)*, 406–428.

Blumer, H. (1969). *Symbolic interactionism: Perspectives and method.* Englewood Cliffs, NJ: Prentice-Hall.

Bohman, J. (1995). Hermeneutics. In R. Audi (Ed.), *The Cambridge dictionary of philosophy* (pp. 323–324). New York: Cambridge University Press.

Bowers, B. J. (1988). Grounded theory. In B. Sarter (Ed.), *Paths to knowledge: Innovative research methods for nursing* (pp. 33–60). Pub. No. 15-2233. New York: National League for Nursing.

Campbell, D. T. (1957). Factors relevant to the validity of experiments in social settings. *Psychological Bulletin, 54(2)*, 297–312.

Campbell, D. T., Fiske, D. W. (1959). Convergent and discriminant validation by the multitrait-multimethod matrix. *Psychological Bulletin, 56(2)*, 81–105.

Cohen, M. Z., & Omery, A. (1994). Schools of phenomenology: Implications for research. In J. M. Morse (Ed.), *Critical issues in qualitative research* (pp. 136–157). Thousand Oaks, CA: Sage.

Darbyshire, P. (1994). Parenting in public: Parental participation and involvement in the care of the hospitalized child. In P. Benner (Ed.), *Interpretive phenomenology: Embodiment, caring, and ethics in health and illness* (pp. 185–210). Thousand Oaks, CA: Sage.

Diekelmann, N. L., Allen, D., & Tanner, C. (1989) *The NLN criteria of appraisal of baccalaureate programs: A critical hermeneutic analysis.* New York: National League for Nursing Press.

Dilthey, W. (1900). The rise of hermeneutics. In P. Connerton (Ed.), *Critical sociology,* 1976 (pp. 106–114). New York: Penguin Books.

Draucker, C. B. (1999a). Knowing what to do: Coping with sexual violence by male intimates. *Qualitative Health Research, 9*(5), 173–484.

Draucker, C. B. (1999b). The critique of Heideggerian hermeneutical nursing research. *Journal of Advanced Nursing, 30*(2), 360–373.

Draucker, C. B., & Madsen, C. (1999). Women dwelling with violence. *Image: Journal of Nursing Scholarship, 31*(9), 327–332.

Draucker, C. B., & Stern, P. N. (2000). Women's responses to sexual violence by male intimates. *Western Journal of Nursing Research, 22*(4), 385–406.

Dreyfus, H. L. (1991). *Being-in-the-world: A commentary on Heidegger's 'Being and Time,' Division I.* Cambridge, MA: MIT Press.

Flick, L. H., & McSweeney, M. (1987). Measures of mother-child interaction: A comparison of three methods. *Research in Nursing & Health, 10*(3), 129–137.

Gadamer, H-G. (1975). *Truth and method.* New York: Seabury Press.

Glaser, B. G. (1978). *Theoretical sensitivity: Advances in the methodology of grounded theory.* Mill Valley, CA: The Sociology Press.

Glaser, B., & Strauss, A. (1967). *The discovery of grounded theory.* Chicago: Aldine.

Goodwin, L. D., & Goodwin, W. L. (1991). Estimating construct validity. *Research in Nursing & Health, 14*(3), 235–243.

Guignon, C. B. (1995). Heidegger. In R. Audi (Ed.), *The Cambridge dictionary of philosophy* (pp. 317–319). New York: Cambridge University Press.

Heidegger, M. (1927/1962). *Being and time.* New York: Harper & Row.

Heidegger, M. (1971). *Poetry, language, and thought* (A. Hofstadter, Trans.). New York: Harper Row.

Knafl, K., Breitmayer, B., Gallo, A., & Zoeller, L. (1992). Parents' views of health care providers: An exploration of the components of a postive working relationship. *Children's Health Care, 21*(2), 90–95.

Koch, T. (1996). Implementation of a hermeneutic inquiry in nursing: Philosophy, rigour, and representation. *Journal of Advanced Nursing, 24,* 174–184.

Makkreel, R. A. (1995). Dilthey. In R. Audi (Ed.). *The Cambridge dictionary of philosophy* (pp. 203–204). New York: Cambridge University Press.

Mead, G. H. (1934/1962). *Mind, self and society: From the standpoint of a social behaviorist.* Chicago: University of Chicago Press.

Morse, J. (1994). Designing funded qualitative studies. In N. K. Denzin & Y. S. Lincoln (Eds.), *Handbook of qualitative research* (pp. 220–235). Thousand Oaks, CA: Sage.

Polkinghorne, D. (1983). *Methodology for the human sciences: Systems of inquiry.* Albany: State University of New York Press.

Ritzer, G. (1983). *Contemporary social theory* (2nd ed.). New York: Alfred A. Knopf.

Stern, P. N. (1994). Eroding grounded theory. In J. M. Morse (Ed.), *Critical issues in qualitative research methods* (pp. 212–223). Thousand Oaks, CA: Sage.

Strauss, A. L., & Corbin, J. (1994). Grounded theory methodology. In N. K. Denzin & Y. S. Lincoln (Eds.), *Handbook of qualitative research* (pp. 273–285). Thousand Oaks, CA: Sage.

Tice, T. N. (1995). Schleiermacher. In R. Audi (Ed.). *The Cambridge dictionary of philosophy* (pp. 716–717). New York: Cambridge University Press.

Van Manen, M. (1990). Research lived experience. Ontario, Canada: Althouse.

Walters, A. J. (1995). A Heideggerian hermeneutic study of the practice of critical care nurses. *Journal of Advanced Nursing, 21,* 492–497.

Welch, D. (1999). Powers of persuasion: Propaganda in the twentieth century. *History Today, 49(8),* 24–26.

Wilson, H. C., & Hutchinson, S. A. (1991). Triangulation of qualitative methods: Heideggerian hermeneutics and grounded theory. *Qualitative Health Research, 1(2),* 263–276.

recognize all participants as European-origin middle-class members of the majority culture unless specified otherwise.

## Interpreting Language Across Research Reports

Closely related to the challenge of elucidating sociocultural context is that of locating and interpreting the language of analyst and participant (Thorne, 1998). Postmodern analysts are attuned to the role of language as arbiter of meaning and power (Denzin, 1994), but we have little guidance as to how verbatim text or analytic labels should be "read" for the purpose of synthesis projects. Noblit and Hare (1988) acknowledged this specifically when they described all research writing as translation, which involves modification of meaning to fit the alternative linguistic paradigm.

When one is attempting to synthesize three clearly linked concepts from three theories into one concept, for example, and each is labeled using a different word with different contextual connotations, how are these influences to be recognized and preserved? In my analysis of studies of women's addiction recovery (Kearney, 1998b), I encountered two studies in which a critical stage of recovery was described as surrendering and a third in which the same juncture was termed transcending denial. Closer examination revealed that the participants from whom the surrender idea had arisen were recruited from (and embedded in the rhetoric of) Alcoholics Anonymous and related twelve-step programs. The transcending denial concept arose from a sample recruited in a psychiatric facility. The language of the participants and their researchers was influenced by these sociocultural contexts. I was required to develop a new description that captured the meanings of both along with concepts from other studies. Only through my past experience studying women in addiction recovery was I sensitized to these standpoints and related linguistic references. Undoubtedly, I failed to understand many other unfamiliar linguistic nuances.

## Discovering the Voice and Influence of the Original Researcher in the Data

Investigators (even postmodern ones) have great power over their participants and the data they provide. It may be impossible to know how a given researcher prompted and elicited particular data from participants during data collection, or how those data were classified and interpreted to serve an unseen theoretical or personal bias. At best, publications include a narrative on the researcher's standpoint and goals that sensitizes readers to a particular shaping and manipulation of data. Otherwise, the formal theorist relies on content, tone, language, coherence, richness, and truth value of data and interpretation to uncover the researcher's implicit standpoint and level of data manipulation. Grounded formal theorists therefore must be interpreters regardless of epistemological stance. Findings do not float free as objective truth independent of their origins (Thorne, 1997). In the synthesis process, during theoretical sampling within and across research reports, during category-building, and during constant comparison of data and theory to derive syntheses of concepts and relationships, one must keep visible the limits and particularities of the contributing material.

## GROUNDED FORMAL THEORY FOR POSTMODERN CLINICIANS

The clinically useful postmodern grounded formal theory is as situated and local as its substantive components. As synthesists we are obliged to clarify our own standpoints, our disciplinary and epistemological perspectives, the points in culture, time, and geography from which we write, and the agendas we hold in seeking and presenting our formal theory. The methods of analysis and synthesis must be described in detail, and the limitations and delimitations of our projects must be clear. The range of variation within the phenomenon must be portrayed in as great a level of complexity as is possible, to do justice to the diverse array of experiences of the pooled participants. And, most important, the findings must have the qualities of good grounded theory (Glaser & Strauss, 1967): they must have fit with the phenomenon, grab the reader with their vivid validity and applicability, work to explain change and variation, and offer insights as to ways of modifying problematic conditions and outcomes.

The clinician reader will ask the same questions of a qualitative synthesis as of any other research report: How much is known, and from what sources? In their scope, perspective, history, and geography, where do these findings sit in relation to other possibilities of experience of this phenomenon? Whose stories are included in the synthesis, and whose are excluded or not yet heard? What is the level of abstraction here, and how do I make this theory concrete in my clinical realm? What are the reasonable clinical applications, and what roads might I be tempted to take in applying these findings that would be clearly unwarranted at this point?

A clinically useful grounded formal theory is not so abstract that its terms seem to float over the realities of illness experience. It is constructed of components that are labeled and linked in recognizable ways and characterize the particularities and diversity of the health or illness experience at hand. Let us avoid "discovering" large hazy words like uncertainty and transformation unless we are prepared to portray in vivid accompanying language the unique kind of uncertainty or transformation this is, the conditions that produce it to differing degrees, and the concrete implications for health meaning and behavior.

Useful formal theory explains some of the more puzzling or challenging problems faced by health care clients and practitioners. Drawing from and generalizing to a situated group of samples, it depicts the personal and situational conditions that contribute to meaning, the components of players' definition of the situation that explain previously unclear behavior, and the range of action and consequences that ensues from these definitions. It maps the possibilities for trajectory of change over time and highlights points of influence open for clinician involvement. It keeps its own boundaries visible. The reader is constantly aware of who is speaking—participant, substantive analyst, or synthesist—and where the speaker is located.

My work has yet to reach this ideal, and many in nursing have struggled to come within reach of the level of rigor that Glaser and Strauss (1967) set out for us. Nurse researchers are pressed by more immediate and different concerns in knowledge development than are medical sociologists. Moreover, what the "founders" set out to achieve was simpler in their more empiricist day than it is in our constructivist time. Nonetheless, grounded formal theory analysis can help nurses raise their substantive inquiry to a higher level of knowledge development, reach across localities to test the common ground of human health experience, and assist patients in reaching common goals. In doing so, it seems wise to expand this theorizing work as far as possible toward the interpretive end of the Meta family continuum. The greater the inclusivity of voices, histories, and geographics in grounded formal theory analyses, the more visible and integrated the standpoints of all whose voices are portrayed; and the more sensitive we are to the language and theoretical origins of the contributing works, as Thorne and Paterson (1998) have demonstrated, the more complete and clinically useful will be the product.

There are few examples or guidelines for this endeavor in nursing—hence, the newly coined labels for newly tried synthesis approaches in the Meta family. Much dialogue and demonstration is needed to refine and strengthen our efforts at grounded formal theory development. The results will look different than those of sociologists or education researchers. Ours in nursing will serve as clinical road maps. As clinicians we will use grounded formal theories to consider possible locations of our patients' experiences in the landscape of experiential variation and identify an array of routes along which we can guide them toward health.

## REFERENCES

Baker Miller, J. (1984). *The development of women's sense of self.* Wellesley, MA: Stone Center for Developmental Services and Studies, Wellesley College.

Barroso, J., & Powell-Cope, G. (2000). Metasynthesis of qualitative research on living with HIV infection. *Qualitative Health Research, 10,* 340–353.

Charmaz, C. (1991). *Good days, bad days: The self in chronic illness and time.* New Brunswick, NJ: Rutgers University Press.

Charmaz, C. (2000). Grounded theory: Objectivist and constructivist methods. In N. Denzin & Y. Lincoln (Eds.), *Handbook of qualitative research,* second edition. Thousand Oaks, CA: Sage.

Clarke, P., Pendry, N., & Kim, Y. (1997). Patterns of violence in homeless women. *Western Journal of Nursing Research, 19,* 490–500.

Corbin, J., & Strauss, A. (1988). *Unending work and care: Managing chronic illness at home.* San Francisco: Jossey-Bass.

Denzin, N. (1994). The art and politics of interpretation. In N. Denzin & Y. Lincoln (Eds.), *Handbook of qualitative research* (pp. 500–515). Thousand Oaks, CA: Sage.

Estabrooks, C., Field, P., & Morse, J. (1994). Aggregating qualitative findings: An approach to theory development. *Qualitative Health Research, 4,* 503–511.

Finfgeld, D. (1999). Courage as a process of pushing beyond the struggle. *Qualitative Health Research, 9,* 803–814.

Fredricksson, L. (1999). Modes of relating in a caring conversation: A research synthesis on presence, touch, and listening. *Journal of Advanced Nursing, 30,* 1167–1176.

Germain, C. (1994). See my abuse: The shelter transition of battered women. In P. Munhall (Ed.), *In women's experience,* vol. 1 (pp. 203–231). New York: National League for Nursing Press.

Gilligan, C. (1982). *In a different voice: Psychological theory and women's development.* Cambridge, MA: Harvard University Press.

Glaser, B. (1968). *Organizational careers: A sourcebook for theory.* Chicago: Aldine.

Glaser, B., & Strauss, A. (1967). *The discovery of grounded theory: Strategies for qualitative research.* New York: Aldine de Gruyter.

Glaser, B., & Strauss, A. (1971). *Status passage: A formal theory.* Chicago: Aldine.

Hilbert, J. (1984). *Pathways of help for battered women: Varying definitions of the situation.* Unpublished dissertation, Case Western Reserve University, Cleveland, OH.

Jensen, L., & Allen, M. (1994). A synthesis of qualitative research in wellness-illness. *Qualitative Health Research, 4,* 349–369.

Jensen, L., & Allen, M. (1996). Meta-synthesis of qualitative findings. *Qualitative Health Research, 6,* 553–560.

Karp, D. (1994). Living with depression: Illness and identity turning points. *Qualitative Health Research, 4,* 6–30.

Kearney, M. H. (1998a). Ready to wear: Discovering grounded formal theory. *Research in Nursing & Health, 21,* 179–186.

Kearney, M. H. (1998b). Truthful self-nurturing: A grounded formal theory of women's addiction recovery. *Qualitative Health Research, 8,* 495–512.

Kearney, M. H. (1999). *Understanding women's recovery from illness and trauma.* Thousand Oaks, CA: Sage.

Kearney, M. H. (2000). Enduring love: A grounded formal theory of women's experience of domestic violence. Manuscript submitted for publication.

Kearney, M. H. (in press). News you can use: Levels and applications of qualitative evidence. *Research in Nursing & Health.*

Kirkevold, M. (1997). Integrative nursing research: An important strategy to further the development of nursing science and nursing practice. *Journal of Advanced Nursing, 25,* 977–984.

Langford, D. (1996). Predicting unpredictability: A model of women's processes of predicting battering men's violence. *Scholarly Inquiry for Nursing Practice, 10,* 371–385.

Langford, D. (1998). Social chaos and danger as context of battered women's lives. *Journal of Family Nursing, 4,* 167–181.

Merritt-Gray, M., & Wuest, J. (1995). Counteracting abuse and breaking free: The process of leaving revealed through women's voices. *Health Care for Women International, 16,* 388–412.

Morse, J., & Johnson, J., Eds. (1991). *The illness experience: Dimensions of suffering.* Newbury Park, CA: Sage.

Noblit, G., & Hare, R. (1988). *Meta-ethnography: Synthesizing qualitative studies.* Newbury Park, CA: Sage.

Sandelowski, M. (1993a). *With child in mind: Studies of the personal encounter with infertility.* Philadelphia: University of Pennsylvania Press.

Sandelowski, M. (1993b). Theory unmasked: The uses and guises of theory in qualitative research. *Research in Nursing & Health, 16,* 213–218.

Sandelowski, M., Docherty, S., & Emden, C. (1997). Qualitative metasynthesis: Issues and techniques. *Research in Nursing & Health, 20,* 365–371.

Schreiber, R., Crooks, D., & Stern, P. N. (1997). Qualitative meta-analysis. In J. Morse (Ed.), *Completing a qualitative project: Details and dialogue* (pp. 311–326). Thousand Oaks, CA: Sage.

Sherwood, G. (1999). Meta-synthesis: Merging qualitative studies to develop nursing knowledge. *International Journal for Human Caring, 3*(1), 37–42.

Thorne, S. (1997). Phenomenological positivism and other problematic trends in health science research. *Qualitative Health Research, 7,* 287–293.

Thorne, S. (1998). Ethical and representational issues in qualitative secondary analysis. *Qualitative Health Research, 8,* 547–555.

Thorne, S., & Paterson, B. (1998). Shifting images of chronic illness. *Image: Journal of Nursing Scholarship, 30,* 173–178.

Wilson, H., & Hutchinson, S. (1996). Methodologic mistakes in grounded theory. *Nursing Research, 45,* 122–124.

Wuest, J. (2000). Negotiating with helping systems: An example of grounded theory evolving through emergent fit. *Qualitative Health Research, 10,* 51–70.

Zhao, S. (1991). Metatheory, metamethod, meta-data-analysis: What, why, and how? *Sociological Perspectives, 34,* 377–390.

# Index